MIND AND BODY IN
EIGHTEENTH CENTURY MEDICINE

MIND AND BODY IN EIGHTEENTH CENTURY MEDICINE

A Study Based on Jerome Gaub's
De regimine mentis

by

L. J. RATHER

UNIVERSITY OF CALIFORNIA PRESS

Berkeley and Los Angeles

1965

Published in the United States of America
by the University of California Press
Berkeley and Los Angeles, California

This work is also published in the United Kingdom
by the Wellcome Historical Medical Library, London

Printed in Great Britain

"... ideas are the beliefs of people, what they assert. They are not, as we use the term, what they would have asserted had they known what we know, or what they should have asserted had they been consistent, or what they might have asserted had they drawn the conclusions from their premises which we would draw."

—George Boas

"Democritus said that if the *sôma* were to enter suit against the *psychê* for cruel and abusive treatment the *psychê* would not be acquitted ... for whenever the *psychê* is preoccupied with its own emotions, strivings and concerns, it is prodigal with the *sôma*."

—Plutarch

"In one set of circumstances the mind is distressed because of a deranged bodily state or, though ailing on its own account, can be healed by remedies acting on the body. In the other the mind causes the bodily disease, or the disease can be suppressed by remedies acting on the mind."

—Jerome Gaub

Table of Contents

Preface

This book offers a new English translation, provided with an introduction, commentaries and notes, of two eighteenth-century essays on the mutual relations of mind and body in health and disease. It has the larger purpose of presenting the reader with a more extensive picture of eighteenth-century psychosomatic medical ideas, based on original sources, than is available in any other book with which I am acquainted. The two essays, first published in the original Latin in the Netherlands in 1747 and 1763, respectively, were the work of Jerome Gaub, professor of medicine and chemistry at the University of Leiden. Only the first essay, translated in the latter part of the eighteenth century by J. Taprell, has hitherto been available in English.

Following the paragraphing of the Latin text I have numbered, grouped and given titles to the paragraphs of my translation, and then embedded the paragraphs in the commentaries. Gaub's first essay deals mainly with his various theses: The inadequacy of current philosophical solutions of the mind-body problem, his views on the physiological mechanism of mind-body interaction, the duty of the physician to care for the whole man, his defense of the physician's concern with the body in connection with mental and emotional disturbances, the nature and variability of the temperaments, the danger of delay in treating the bodily cause of a mental ailment, the need for a concerted search by physicians for new drugs capable of affecting the mind, and some others. The second essay treats in more conventional eighteenth-century fashion of the harmful and beneficial effects of the emotions on the body in health and disease, and of the therapeutic use of the emotions. The commentary and notes on the second essay present the beliefs of a number of Gaub's contemporaries and forebears, and take an occasional forward glance toward the present.

Western medicine, from its origins in the Greek world of the fifth century before our era down to the present day, has never ceased to grapple with the problem of assessing the relative importance of mental and physical factors in the causation and treatment of ailments of the body and mind. Diet, drugs and surgery are the traditional measures against ailments of the body. To what extent are they applicable to ailments of the mind, to disturbances of the emotions? The word—the chief medium of exchange of human meaning—is the traditional measure against mental or emotional disturbances. To what extent is this measure applicable to ailments of the body? To what extent are mental and emotional disturbances effective in producing or curing bodily ailments, to what extent are they the results of bodily derangements? That these questions are part of the tradition of Western medicine has been lost sight of in recent times. For this reason developments in the field of psychosomatic medicine in our own day have had the flavor of complete novelty for many. The present book aims to show something of the extent to which the question of the relation of body to mind in human ailments, both mental and physical, is one of the perennial topics of Western thought.

The reader should perhaps be warned in advance that I am not concerned here with the truth value, in the light of present-day beliefs, of the material presented. Aquinas is said to have remarked that the legitimate aim of philosophy is not to know what men have thought but to ascertain how the truth of the matter stands. This is also the legitimate aim of natural science. But it should not be taken as the sole aim of the history of science and still less as that of the history of medicine. We may with some justice say rather that the aim of the history of medicine *is* to know what men have thought. Nor is this the simple matter that it may appear to be on first sight. We may be required in so doing to regard with sympathetic eyes a way of comprehending the world or some of its aspects that is very different from our own. And even when our own tradition is the subject of our study we may run into difficulties that recall those confronting the anthropologist in his attempt to grasp the medical thought of some primitive or isolated tribe without imposing on it his own concepts and beliefs. The positivistic historian of science and medicine, following in the wake of the triumphant modern scientist, has often been so certain of the truth that he has found it difficult in consequence to accord his forebears the courtesy of careful and unprejudiced study. One of the besetting sins of the scientific present has frequently been a certain contempt and lack of understanding for the scientific past. Yet we find often enough that when men have made what they believe to be radical intellectual departures from the past they have in fact done little more than resurrect or reshuffle older beliefs. The familiar saying that those who do not understand history are condemned to repeat it is more relevant in connection with intellectual history than anywhere else.

I wish to express my thanks to Stanford University for granting me a sabbatical year in 1962–63, during which a major part of this book was written, and to the National Institutes of Health for partial financial support during that and previous years. I am grateful to Professor Dr. Werner Leibbrand for allowing me access to the Heinrich Laehr collection of books on neurology and psychiatry in the *Institut der Geschichte der Medizin* of the University of Munich during my sabbatical year. I am grateful also for the many courtesies extended me by the staff of the Wellcome Historical Medical Library in London, by the staff of the History of Medicine Division of the National Library of Medicine in Washington, D.C., and by Miss Clara Manson, Mrs. Anna Hoen and the staff of the Lane Medical Library of the Stanford University School of Medicine. I thank my secretary, Mrs. Ulla Noor Warner, for her hours of painstaking work on a difficult manuscript. I am indebted to Dr. Saul Jarcho for some helpful comments on parts of the translation. My greatest debt of thanks I owe to my friend Dr. John B. Frerichs. He reviewed the entire translation in connection with the original Latin text, and carefully read and criticized the commentaries, notes and appendices as well. Any errors that may remain are my own.

Introduction

1. *The Mind-Body Problem in Medical Thought*

In their concern with the cause, cure, nature, prognosis and meaning of human illness the thoughts of men in general and physicians in particular have revolved around a small number of themes. Of these themes that of the relation between mind and body in health and disease—involving as it does the question of the proper role of the physician in treating mental and emotional disturbances, and of the extent to which emotional disturbances produce structural and functional changes in the body—is among the most important. To the non-medical student of ideas it is also one of the most interesting of these themes, since it transcends the narrow limits of medicine as a specialized technique and is part of the more general problem of the nature of man.

As far as the discipline of medicine is concerned, the theme of the relation between mind and body in health and disease is not precisely identical with the perennial mind-body problem that has so greatly troubled philosophers during the past three hundred years or more. Medical theorists and, still less, practicing physicians have not regarded it as their business throughout this time to unite the philosophical categories of mind and body, the disparity of which was so convincingly set forth to his contemporaries by Descartes. It seemed plain to most of them that the will and the emotions did in one way or another produce far-reaching and sometimes harmful or even fatal changes in the body, and they believed it their business as physicians to set forth the circumstances, extent and means of control of the interaction between mind and body. They believed also, in keeping with an unbroken tradition originating in ancient Greek medicine, that the mind could be influenced corporeally, that is, by means of drugs, diet, climate and other factors acting primarily on the body. Clinical observation had convinced them that the cause of a bodily disturbance could lie in the mind, and that where this was so treatment of the body alone was sometimes ineffectual. On the other hand, it had also convinced them that the causes of some mental disorders lay in the body, and they drew the obvious inference regarding treatment.

The philosophical—as distinguished from the physiological—question at issue in disputes over the role that psychic factors play in the initiation of somatic disease is the question of how they can act as causes in physical systems. How is it possible, given certain other accepted beliefs, to conceive of this? The question is not a purely empirical one, since certain requirements of theory must be satisfied when the empirical evidence is interpreted. To put it another way, the parties to the dispute hold presuppositions that make certain interpretations of the evidence objectionable. Nothing purporting to show that mental or emotional stress can cause fever, stomach ulcers, skin rashes (or, to borrow from the eighteenth century, contribute to the onset of contagious disease) will, for example, convince someone already committed to the belief that ulcers, rashes, and so forth are events in the physical world and therefore *must* ultimately have physicochemical causes. If we replace "cause", with its anthropomorphic overtones, by "determining antecedent events" the position of the skeptic becomes clear. He will hold that these determining antecedent events are and *must* be physicochemical events subject to the same natural laws regardless of whether they take place inside or outside of the human skin.

For this reason he will be unimpressed by the next move in the gambit most often adopted by the proponent of the psychic (or psychological, as is more commonly and euphemistically said) causation of disease. This is to admit that the ulcer or rash is not directly caused by an emotional disturbance or by anything else of "mental" character. These effects, so the argument goes, are the end result of a long chain of events linking together the brain, peripheral nervous system and endocrine glands with the ultimate fine structure and function of the cells and tissues in such a way as to cause the bodily damage in question. The visible structural changes (skin rash or ulcer) are the result of functional changes that, in turn, are brought about by nerve impulses taking their origin in subcortical centers of the brain, where the emotions (or rather their neurophysiological counterparts) are thought to be localized.

The skeptic rightly replies that this is merely to transform the mind-body problem into the mind-brain problem. "You are", we can hear him say, "trying to hide the stumbling block of interaction in the recesses of the brain. How can emotional disturbances—meaning neither their neurophysiological counterparts nor the objectively observable behavior of the person concerned, but the raw experiences themselves—discharge neurones any more than they can directly cause ulcers?"[1] Our skeptic holds that physical reality is all of reality and that human beings are no more than immensely complicated physicochemical machines. Not simply man's body—those "hydraulico-pneumatical engines we call human bodies", as Robert Boyle remarked, in the middle of the seventeenth century[2]— but *man himself* is such a machine, so he believes. Physicochemical events can have physicochemical antecedent determining events only. How then can conscious (or unconscious) disturbances of the mind possibly initiate functional or structural changes in the body? Is it not clearly illegitimate—and physically impossible—to introduce anything mental or psychic into the bodily machinery as an effective force no matter how small the quantum of force is taken to be?

Within the framework of post-Cartesian beliefs about mind and body the skeptic's position is quite sound, even if we admit the occurrence of psychokinesis. Attempts have been repeatedly made, from Descartes on down to the present day, to introduce mind as an effective agent into a neurophysiological chain of events. To mention only the most recent of these: A well-known neurophysiologist states that

3

we must assume freedom of the will if our activities as scientific investigators are to make any sense at all. Yet, he continues, if the will is able to modify our reactions in any given situation it can do so only by influencing the pattern of neuronal activity in the brain, and this perhaps by exerting a weak spatiotemporal field of influence detected and amplified by the cerebral cortex, possibly from below the level of intensity so far accessible to physical instrumentation.[3] Such a proposal, like its many predecessors, remains within the circle of Cartesian neurophysiology. It posits psychokinesis, a direct effect of mind on matter. While "internal" psychokinesis is accepted by most people without question before they begin to philosophize, as Descartes remarked in different words on one occasion,[4] "external" psychokinesis, although vouched for by writers from Avicenna to J. B. Rhine, is not quite respectable. The mind is usually accorded a considerable degree of dominance within the body, but is regarded as quite powerless without.[5] Let us suppose, however, that at some future time it will have been shown to everyone's satisfaction that both internal and external psychokinesis actually occur. Not only can the mind affect its body (or its brain) but it can directly affect the external material world: For example, the fall of a die will have been conclusively proven to have been influenced by the will of the thrower. A moment's thought will show that the status of the mind-body problem will remain essentially unchanged. Either we shall then be able to prove that some hitherto unknown physical agency associated with the brain is producing these changes in the material world or we shall not. If so, the puzzle of the relation between willing and the physical agency will replace the puzzle of the relation between willing and the discharge of a cerebral neuron or between willing and the fall of the die. If not, the dilemma in its original form will remain. In other words, the problem is not likely to be resolved within the set of presuppositions that helped generate it.

The mind-body dilemma is nevertheless a genuine one

4

and no mere consequence of the incorrect use of words. It arises partly as the result of a certain set of beliefs about the nature of reality, and for this reason it has become acute in a definite historical setting. While an escape from its horns may yet be possible, the failure of three hundred years of intellectual tauromachy to achieve one that satisfies all parties should make us wary of attempts to do so with a few phrases.[6] The structure of modern science, it has been said, was built up largely on the basis of the Cartesian distinction of the mental from the physical. The subjective observer was partially excluded in this effort.[7] Few of the opponents of dualism have given proper recognition to the likelihood that an equally gigantic effort might be required to reconstruct the edifice of science after introducing the subject. Changing the metaphor, to repair the "flaw in the great diamond" (as Merleau-Ponty has called it), the flaw in the picture of the world that we ourselves are, the perceiving subjects through whom that world comes into existence, may prove to be no easy task.[8]

Descartes' rediscovery of and emphasis on the primacy of awareness was, after all, a fundamental insight. To illustrate one of its most crucial aspects let us suppose ourselves presented with a humanoid computer able to reproduce every nuance of behavior that could be used to distinguish a man from a machine. To distinguish the machine from what had hitherto been called a man would be a simple matter, since it would, presumably, consist of transistors and wires rather than cells and fibers. Our machine will converse learnedly in any tongue, it will compose music, write scholarly books if given access to libraries, utter convincing views regarding the mind-body problem, and complain of discomfort when one of its parts functions improperly. In short, no criterion will remain to distinguish the behavior of this automaton from that of a human being. Is it not true, the constructor of the machine may ask, that there is no need whatsoever to posit "mind" as a ghost in this machine and hence, by analogy, no reason to posit mind in the human body or brain? One may say, if one wishes, that a mind is embodied in the first instance in the form of transistors and wires, in the second in the less tidy framework of the human body, but is not "mind", as a real existent at least, an unnecessary and ultimately confusing assumption? Why not accept the reduction of "mind" to mind-like physical behavior? We may have one further question. Is the machine aware as we are aware, does it have the experience of interior life as we experience it? A nonsensical because forever unverifiable question, retorts the constructor. He is joined at this point by a behavioristic psychologist who assures us that everything human can be reduced to objective behavior. The question does nevertheless make sense, because each one of us knows very well what is meant, whether or not there is any way of finding out if the automaton does. To try to resolve the mind-body problem by eliminating the subject—for this is what "mind" has meant since Descartes—is a favorite maneuver but no solution. Yet there is no denying that this observer, this "ghost in the machine" that Ryle[9] has recently attempted to exorcize, is in a highly precarious position within the spatio-temporal world of physical science. There is literally no place for that observer who is each of us unless he is transformed into an aspect of a mechanism the workings of which have somehow acquired the puzzling feature of "awareness". But the transformation cannot be allowed, for we can no more extrapolate to "awareness" in a machine than we can slip in mind as an efficient cause in a physical system. As William James remarked here, you cannot excuse the presence of an illegitimate infant with the plea that it is a very small one.[10]

It is obvious that the billiard-ball universe of nineteenth-century mechanistic materialism had no place for such an insubstantial entity as mind. It is perhaps less obvious that the flaw in the great diamond has not been repaired by the reconstructive work of physicists in our own time. Heisenberg's uncertainty principle has no bearing whatsoever on the problem of free will, and the observer of Einsteinian physics could equally well be an electronic device.

6

The chasm lying between subject and object remains as great as it ever was, and in the background of the world picture of triumphant physical science what Berkeley called the "perceiving active being", the "mind", "soul", "spirit", the "I myself" persists, mocking the completeness of the picture but fitting into the new universe of physics no better than into the older one.

Let us return for a moment to the medical aspect of the mind-body problem. We have previously noted the long-standing belief of Western physicians that the mind and the emotions had something to do with ailments of the body. What are the medical sources of this belief? We may approach the answer to this question by examining first the deliverance of unreflective thought, before it has been subjected to the demands of a theoretical system that admits certain events and dismisses others as impossible. This naïve attitude of unreflective thought gave rise at an early date in the development of our culture to the belief that our "feelings"—love, hate, hope, fear, and so on—are, when followed by changes in the body, responsible for those changes. I smile because I am happy, I blush because I am ashamed. The various "emotions"—however they may be parcelled out and designated—are thought to bring about characteristic changes in the external appearance of the body. Nothing seems more obvious. The possibility that corresponding internal changes in the body ensue requires little exercise of the imagination or further observation. The only problems arising at this stage are empirical ones, such as the determination of just what does happen in the body in particular circumstances, the nature of intermediate or difficultly observable events, and so on.

The philosophical problem arises when mind and body are ontologically sundered and assigned to two different realms of being. Not the details of the physiological mechanism of mind-body interaction, however intricate and puzzling they may be, are then at issue, but the very possibility of interaction itself. Descartes is usually credited with carrying out the split, yet it is perfectly plain that a

7

philosophical and theological mind-body (or soul-body) problem is deeply embedded in the Platonic-Augustinian tradition and that Descartes's achievement was to state the problem clearly and distinctly at a crucial time in the development of Western thought. Even in medical circles, prior to Descartes, there was some puzzlement over the possibility of mind-body interaction. This can be seen from Thomas Wright's comment in a book published more than fifty years before Descartes wrote, that while physicians agree that strong emotions alter the four humors of the body and that among the various extrinsic causes of disease emotional excess is not one of the least, it busies both their brains and those of natural philosophers to explain "how an operation lodged in the soul or mind can alter the body and move its corporeal humors from place to place".[11] And Descartes's solution? The familiar scheme of inter-action of mind and body at the site of the pineal gland is a physiological hypothesis, not a philosophical explanation. The truth is that, when pushed into a corner, he had none. Writing to Princess Elisabeth of Bohemia in 1643 Descartes advised her that the union of mind and body could be under-stood only in terms of everyday life. The princess had repeatedly pressed him for a solution to the problem of how two things so utterly disparate as mind and body could act on each other. The philosopher replied that mind, *res cogitans*, could be grasped only by the pure intellect, and matter, *res extensa*, by the intellect with the aid of the imagination. But the mode of union of the two could be understood only by means of sense experience in daily life. It was for this reason, Descartes assured her, that men who were not philosophers had no doubt whatsoever that mind and body acted on each other in turn. And we shall see that when Descartes himself discusses the effects of the emotions on bodily health he reverts to the traditional view and tacitly allows efficacy to the emotions.[12]

Descartes's escape into the realm of immediate experience from a mind-body dilemma generated by his own strict dualism recalls David Hume's equally well-known flight to the bosom of his friends—"determined to live and talk, and act like other people in the common affairs of life"—to escape the uncomfortable consequences of his own skeptical philosophy.[13] An escape-hatch into the world of immediate experience is opened and both philosophers climb through to resume intercourse with human beings like themselves. A phenomenologist would perhaps say that they re-enter the *Lebenswelt*. If it is the right and duty of some philosophers to withdraw from the world of direct experience to work out the ultimate theoretical consequences of their assumptions, it is equally the right and duty of other philosophers to point out—as the phenomenologists have been doing lately—that the starting point of any philosophical flight is always our immediate "lived" experience. How to be certain that we are making contact with immediate experience, disguised as it often is by a welter of beliefs, presuppositions and theoretical constructs, is another matter, nor is it clear what we are to do with a scientific structure reared on the basis of an abstraction from lived experience.

Somewhat similar relations obtain between the medical theorist and the practicing physician. The latter is aware that he treats neither minds nor bodies in isolation. He treats people whom he takes to be more or less like himself. And he knows that the way these people feel about themselves, their physician, their treatment, and their immediate human environment may have important effects on their bodily ailments. The practicing physician soon finds that he cannot behave like the philosopher and ignore the world of "lived" experience in favor of a theoretical construct. His patients are unwilling to permit this, and insofar as he is a genuine therapist he will be disinclined to do so.

It is perhaps for this reason that a strain of psychosomatic practice runs through Western medicine, even though Western medical theory has been concerned largely with the body. To be sure, this therapeutic tradition has often been overshadowed by the growth and power of medical theories placing exclusive weight on corporeal phenomena.

9

Here, perhaps, lies part of the meaning of the often repeated stories, attached to such great medical names as Hippocrates and Galen, in which the cause of a puzzling illness is diagnosed by the physician shrewd and knowledgeable enough to observe the bodily effects of longing and unsatisfied desires—whose finger is on the pulse of a person rather than on that of a physiological machine.[14] "Woe to the medical man", wrote the French physician Cabanis in 1795, "who has not learned to read the human heart as well as to recognize the febrile state! ... How can he restore calm to the disturbed spirit, to the mind consumed by persistent melancholy if he ignores those organic lesions which such moral disorders can cause and the functional disorders with which they are connected?"[15] And Jerome Gaub tells us that while the physician is "mentally able to abstract body from mind and consider it separately in order to be less confused in the marshalling of his ideas", in practice "where he deals with man as he is, should he devote all his efforts to the body alone, and take no account of the mind, his curative efforts will pretty often be less than happy", for "the reason why a sound body becomes ill or an ailing body recovers may lie in the mind. Contrariwise the body frequently both begets mental illnesses and heals its offspring."[16]

2. *Jerome Gaub's Views on Psychosomatic Medicine, and their Relationship to the Medical Tradition*

The reader may ask if it is permissible to apply the term —some will say the catchword—psychosomatic medicine to the content of Gaub's two discourses on the medical management of the mind. If the employment of depth psychology or psychoanalysis in the investigation or treatment of the conditions in question is meant the answer is, of course, no. But the answer is yes if we mean the study of the relationship of emotions to bodily changes in health and disease, if we mean the claim that the causes of some diseases of the body can be traced to disturbances of the mind or emotions, and, finally, if we mean the thesis that mind and body are abstractions from man as he actually exists.

Gaub begins the first of his two discourses with a brief treatment of current philosophical theories regarding the relationship between mind and body. He rejects theories that conceive of the mind as a prisoner in the body or as a "god in a machine" on the grounds that the power of the mind over the body is either overlooked on the one hand or exaggerated on the other. Furthermore, he considers that to regard the mind as all-powerful in the body fails to take proper account of the many involuntary bodily activities familiar to every physician. Gaub's espousal of the evidence of direct experience becomes plain in connection with his refusal to accept Leibnizian psycho-physical parallelism. He devotes considerable time to an exposition of the solution of the mind-body dilemma offered by Leibniz, but ends by calling it a "fable whose novelty has recommended it, whose recommendation has spread it, whose spread has polished it, refined and finally adorned it with . . . a pleasing look of truth", and asks how anyone can accept something so at variance with the results of self-observation. "I appeal", he continues, "to your inner awareness, the testimony of which, with all due restrictions, ought to be given major consideration in this matter".[17] We cannot fail to comment that Gaub does not do justice to the subtleties of Leibniz' argument. Given the utterly disparate features of the Cartesian *res cogitans* and *res extensa*, given the law of the conservation of force, the interaction of mind and body seemed impossible to Leibniz. His doctrine of psycho-physical parallelism on the basis of a pre-established harmony really is a brilliant solution of the dilemma. But, as Gaub saw, it is no less unconvincing than it is irrefutable. Gaub then, like many physicians before him, tells his auditors that they must not expect him to expound the nature of the relation between mind and body, for he neither understands it himself nor has he any hope that man will ever understand it. He will not "invent something new and seemingly more appropriate to embellish what cannot be explained."[18]

Gaub holds that the physician should intervene in the management of mind-body interrelations in two sets of circumstances. On the one hand the mental disturbance may be due to a deranged condition of the body, or, even though not primarily due to a bodily disturbance, can best be treated by measures taken against the body. On the other hand the mind may cause bodily disease, or, though the causes of the disease lie primarily in the body, remedies acting on the mind may beneficially affect its course. He admits that the care of the mind is chiefly the concern of the philosopher, and he proposes therefore to limit himself to circumstances in which the body dominates the mind. To a limited degree it is within the power of the physician to modify the bodily temperament and thereby control the mind. He may do this by employing agents acting directly on the body or by removing agents that are influencing the body. A drunkard, Gaub tells us, is best controlled by withdrawing alcohol (corporeal therapy) rather than by inculcating moral precepts during his sober moments in the hope of improving his behavior during subsequent episodes of inebriety (therapy of the mind). Suggesting that physicians should pay more attention to the treatment of mental derangement by means of drugs and physical shock, Gaub asks also that they consider more seriously the possible effects of subtle bodily changes on mental states. When the mental disturbance is associated with some obvious bodily change—here he cites various kinds of abnormal behavior observed during pregnancy—the need for the services of the physician is plain to everyone. But the bodily cause of a mental disturbance need not be immediately obvious, and he holds that physicians should give more attention to this possibility.

Paradoxical as it may seem to the reader brought up in the belief that modern psychosomatic medicine represents a radical departure from medical thought of the past, it was not Gaub's emphasis on the psychological factors in the causation of disease that surprised and disturbed some of his contemporaries. It was rather the degree of stress that he placed on the need for obtaining additional means to control the mind by means of agents acting on the body. He described the few drugs available in his time effective in this respect and called on physicians to throw themselves wholeheartedly into the investigation of this neglected aspect of the art of medicine. In doing so he moved on dangerous ground. By emphasizing the bodily mechanisms controlling the mind or soul he might seem both to take away from the importance of the soul and to enter into conflict with the religious doctrine of free will. While it was perfectly acceptable and usual in his time to regard man's *body* as a machine, an increasing emphasis on the subordination of mind to body would threaten to reduce *man* to a machine. This was, of course, far from acceptable. Julien La Mettrie, a physician, and like Gaub a pupil of the great clinician Hermann Boerhaave, made just this reduction. His *succès de scandale*, *Man a Machine*, was published somewhat less than a year after 8 February 1747, the date on which Gaub delivered his first essay as a public lecture. La Mettrie not only attended this lecture (where Gaub observed him) but made use of some of the illustrative material for his own purposes. This was a source of embarrassment to Gaub, as we know from one of his letters to the Swiss psychologist, Charles Bonnet. It made him, he wrote to Bonnet, more cautious in dealing with the subject in his textbook (the *Institutiones Pathologiae Medicinalis*) and also led him to preface his second essay with a short diatribe against La Mettrie and a justification of his remarks on the previous occasion.[19]

The second essay was designed to cover that aspect of the mind-body relationship in which mind is the determining factor in bodily disease. In conventional eighteenth-century fashion Gaub takes up one emotion after another, discussing their bodily effects and their roles in the cause and cure of ailments of the body. He deals also with the problem of the natural restoration of physiological balance and the role of the healing power of nature—a perennial topic in medicine since the days of Hippocrates—and seeks for the shadowy boundary line between the psychological and the physiological aspects of man. Toward the end of the essay he reverts once again to his earlier thesis, pointing out that the physician is often unable to "govern the mind by means of the mind itself", that is, with words, and in consequence may find it necessary to govern the mind indirectly through action taken against the body, that is, by drugs and physical measures.

One of Gaub's sources was Galen's study of the relationship of bodily temperament to human behavior, familiar to him in its Latin version, *Quod animi mores corporis temperamenta sequantur*.[20] This study, written in the second century of our era by one of the two most influential of the ancient physicians, can conveniently be taken to mark the start of a long search for means to control the mind and human behavior with agents acting on the body that is still being pursued with great enthusiasm (but perhaps less understanding) in our own time. Another of Gaub's sources is to be found in Cicero, in particular that section of the Tusculan Disputations dealing with the emotions. Finally, the writings of Descartes influenced Gaub, although perhaps to a lesser degree than might be expected. Descartes's claim (made in the Discourse on Method) that only in the art of medicine will we find means to improve mankind "since the spirit depends so greatly on the temperament and the state of the bodily organs", echoes Galen. Gaub quotes the claim with approval in his first essay.[21] The influence exerted by the temperament, that is, by the varying constitution of the *body*, on mind or soul had long since become a medical commonplace and the title of Galen's above-mentioned essay a medical proverb. But now physicians were being called upon to take action in the light of these frequently quoted words.

Gaub's theory of the emotions and bodily changes remained within the dominant medical tradition and did not follow the new path marked out a century before by Descartes. That is to say, Gaub regards an emotion first and foremost as a disturbance of the *mind*. The disturbance is

14

then transmitted to the body, where it gives rise to characteristic effects, harmful or beneficial depending on the circumstances. Descartes, on the other hand, regarded emotions chiefly as disturbances or, better, as readjustments of the *bodily* mechanism set off by external stimuli with the physiological aim of readying the body for flight or defense. The subtle distinctions drawn between body and mind in *Les Passions de l'Âme* conflicted with the medical tradition and were either not fully understood or ignored by both Gaub and most of his medical contemporaries. Physicians continued to attribute to the intervention of mind in bodily processes much that Descartes himself would have ascribed to the working of the bodily mechanism alone, allowing the mind little more than an awareness of the corporeal events taking place.

It has perhaps already been made sufficiently plain to the reader that Gaub was not a pioneer in the field of what is now called psychosomatic medicine. For the most part he said nothing that hundreds of physicians had not said before him. The triumph celebrated by somatic medicine —medicine centering almost exclusively on the body as an object of scientific study—in the nineteenth century, and in particular the importance achieved by pathological anatomy in the new form of cellular pathology, to a very great degree succeeded in wiping out recollection of the attention traditionally accorded to mind-body relationships. Hence psychosomatic medicine in our time has appeared to many as a new and almost unprecedented movement in medical thought. In order to place Gaub somewhat more firmly within the intellectual context of his time a few additional remarks will be made regarding the Western medical tradition.

There is much to be said for the view, put forward by the Spanish historian and philosopher of medicine, Pedro Lain-Entralgo, that Western medicine and the Greek medicine on which it is based are radically naturalistic, overemphasizing the role of the body and slighting that of the *person*.[22] The one-sided emphasis of Greek medicine was already the subject of criticism in Plato's time.[23]　However, this does not mean that the Greeks wholly ignored the psychological aspect of bodily disease.　Lain-Entralgo points out that the term "psychosomatic medicine" may mean one of two things today—either an elaboration and attempted union of the more or less traditional psychological and somatic trends in Western medicine, originating with the Greeks and extending down to modern times, or a view of disease in which the sick man is first and foremost a free person.　In keeping with the distinction drawn by Lain-Entralgo, I emphasize here that the background of "psychosomatic medicine" in which Gaub's work appears must be viewed under the first heading.　In Gaub, too, we can see a bias, characteristic of Western medicine and especially evident today, toward the transformation of moral into physiological problems.　Attention is called to this bias here for the purpose, not of wholesale condemnation, but of recognition and evaluation.

It was Galen, too, who pointed out that physicians were often baffled by ailments because they failed to realize the extent to which the *psyche* could affect the *soma*.[24]　In many places in his works Galen calls attention to the effects of the emotions on the body, and he specifically includes the emotions among the causes of bodily disease.[25]　Latin versions of the medical works of writers in Arabic re-introduced Galen's ideas into the European medical tradition in the twelfth century after a long slow circuit through Byzantium, Syria, Persia, North Africa and southern Italy. The doctrine of pertinence to us here, that of the six "non-naturals", made its European début in the Isagoge of Joannitius, a Latin translation of a commentary on Galen's *Ars parva* by ibn Ishāq.　The "non-naturals" originate in Galen as six categories of causes important in determining disease or health.　The sixth of these includes what we today call "emotions".[26]

In spite of the advances in anatomy and physiology made since the twelfth century—especially since the sixteenth century—physicians of Gaub's day still held to some aspects of the Galenical tradition of medical treatment with great persistence. Down to the end of the eighteenth century they continued to write books, monographs and dissertations on the six non-naturals, devoting considerable attention to the sixth of these, the affections, perturbations, emotions or passions of the mind.[27] On the whole Gaub's contemporaries ascribed as much or more in the way of bodily change to the emotions or "power of the imagination" than would all but the most convinced proponents of the psychological causation of disease today. Not only were the antecedent causes of many derangements of the body thought to lie in the mind but, more specifically, emotional states were believed to influence susceptibility to certain contagious and epidemic diseases and even to influence the clinical course of cancer (the latter claim, incidentally, has been recently revived). Thus we see that Gaub's two essays on mind-body relationships of concern to the physician were quite as much within the medical tradition as would have been essays on the role of diet or climate (which were also among the "non-naturals") in the management of bodily illness. It was not until the nineteenth century, and then only gradually and incompletely, that textbooks of general medicine began to dispense with discussions of the emotions in connection with the cause and cure of ailments of the body.

3. Jerome Gaub's Life and Work

The reader has by now perhaps developed enough interest in Jerome Gaub to welcome a brief account of his life and work. The following, based mainly on secondary contemporary sources, makes no pretense at completeness. A full scale biography has not been written in any language, to my knowledge.

Gaub was a man of considerable stature in the world of medicine. That he was known throughout Europe and Great Britain both the multitude of learned societies to which he belonged and the frequent citation of his opinions by contemporary writers attest. He was a member of the Royal Society of London, of the Society of Experimental Philosophy of Rotterdam, of the Academy of Science of Haarlem, of the Academy of Science and Belles-Lettres of the Palatine Elector of Mannheim, of the Royal Society of Medicine at Paris, and of learned societies in Zeeland, Edinburgh and St. Petersburg, at the time of his death on 29 November 1780.[28] His fame as professor of medicine and chemistry at the University of Leiden was such that the Empress Elizabeth of Russia made repeated attempts to recruit him as her chief physician, even going so far as to enlist the services of Abraham Kaau-Boerhaave in an effort to persuade Gaub's wife of the honors awaiting her husband at the Russian court.[29] Her successor on the throne, Catherine the Great, is also said to have singled him out with marks of favor.[30] Gaub preferred, however, to remain in Leiden as the leading figure at the medical school. There he was three times chosen Rector. Evidence of the esteem Gaub enjoyed in Holland is that, although he was a foreigner, the Estates-General gave him the post of chief physician to William V, Prince of Orange, when it fell vacant in 1760 (the Prince being then still in his minority).[31] Some of the men who studied under Gaub at Leiden went on to occupy professorial chairs in universities in Holland and Germany. Gaub himself remained in his chair until seventy, when his activities began to be interrupted by frequent attacks of gout.[32] His death at the age of seventy-five was unexpected, since he had been by no means mentally and physically moribund up until the final episode, an acute and rapidly fatal fever.[33]

Jerome David Gaub was born in Heidelberg on 24 February 1705, the son of Christoph Gaub and the grandson of Johann Kaspar Gaub. The latter had been a cavalry colonel in the wars of the Palatinate that had left much of Heidelberg in ruins in 1693. Christoph Gaub, according to his son's French eulogist, was a small manufacturer who joined in the efforts of his fellow townspeople to cause the town to rise again from the ashes.[34] Although a Protestant,

Christoph Gaub confided the early education of his son to the Jesuits. Jerome was so warmly received and cared for at the Jesuit school that his father began to fear a design to convert the boy, and he resolved therefore to place him elsewhere.[35]

Shortly before this time August Hermann Francke (1663–1727), a well-known pietist, pedagogue and Protestant divine who was professor of theology at the University of Halle, had established a school and home for outcast and orphaned children. It was this school to which Christoph Gaub dispatched his son. In 1698 there were one hundred orphans and five hundred day scholars under Francke's charge.[36] These schools, bearing the designation of *Francke'sche Stiftungen*, have persisted down to modern times. In Gaub's day the curriculum is said to have been strictly religious, emphasizing Hebrew and neglecting the Greek and Latin classics.[37] Gaub's French eulogist deals rather harshly with the program of studies and general conduct of the school, calling it "pedantry reinforced by ignorance and fanaticism".[38] It seems that Gaub and Francke became equally dissatisfied with each other, and the boy was returned to his father with the suggestion from Francke that he be directed toward some non-intellectual pursuit. He was nevertheless sent away to study again, this time in the care of his uncle, Joan Gaub, a well-known physician of Amsterdam.[39]

Jerome is said to have acquired a taste for medical studies from his uncle. He began to study medicine formally, first under Bartholomew de Moor in Harderwyk and afterwards under Hermann Boerhaave at Leiden. He took his degree at Leiden in 1725 with an inaugural dissertation on the solid parts of the human body.[40] The eulogist, and, following him, Gruner, say that this dissertation already indicates his disinclination toward the systems of the iatromechanicians.[41] The basis for this statement is not plainly evident. Gaub refers to the body as an hydraulic machine without objecting to this designation,[42] and although he reminds his readers that an *animus* (mind) is

19

present throughout the machine[43] we can hardly regard this as a tenet unacceptable to all iatromechanicians. The dissertation concerns itself with the problem of the fundamental unit of structure of the human body. Gaub defines an "element" as the simplest unit of matter from which mixed bodies are constituted. He then mentions briefly the atoms of Democritus, the four elements of the Peripatetics, the two element view derived from the latter (i.e. that fire and water suffice), the three elements of the "adepts" (salt, sulfur and mercury), and the claim of "more recent chemists" that water and earth are the true elementary substances. The latter hold, he says, that human bodies are composed of water, spirit, volatile salt, oil and earth, and that fire will resolve any solid part of any animal into these components (most of which are modifications of earth).[44] However, this does not answer the question with which he is concerned, namely, what is the element, the matter, responsible for the texture of the solid parts of the body?[45] The basis of the solid parts of our bodies, he replies, is pure, simple, elementary earth, the earth of the chemists, and he quotes Boerhaave's definition of this substance.[46] The linear union of these cohesive atomic particles generates the elementary fibers of animal bodies.[47]

After receiving his degree in medicine at Leiden Gaub left Holland for France, where he spent a year in study, busying himself with anatomy, surgery and obstetrics.[48] He then revisited Heidelberg, but returned to Holland within a very short time—drawn back, according to the eulogist, by his attraction for his cousin-german, Constantia, the daughter of Joan Gaubius.[49] In 1726 we find him established as city-physician, under the direction of his uncle, in Deventer.[50] He is said to have occupied himself with the study of pharmacy during this time.[51] The outbreak of an epidemic of fever in Amsterdam in 1727 brought him back to that city, and he spent the next two years aiding in the attempt to check the disease.[52]

Boerhaave, who had not lost sight of him, was at this time sixty-two years old and desirous of some relief from his heavy duties as a teacher. At his request Gaub was called to the University of Leiden as lecturer in chemistry (*Lector chemiae*) on 21 May 1731,[53] and van Royen was at the same time appointed lecturer in botany, thus relieving Boerhaave of two of his posts.[54] Gaub's inaugural oration dealt with a justification of the inclusion of chemistry among the academic disciplines.[55] A revealing insight into Gaub's professional character can be found in one of his letters to Albrecht Haller. Gaub recounts the events of his life after 1726 and remarks that his appointment as lecturer in chemistry had relieved him of the tedium of medical practice, to which he was "most ill suited".[56] A few testimonials to his ability as a teacher are available. One contemporary speaks of his clear and methodical presentations,[57] another of his experimental demonstrations,[58] and the chief regret of a third is that he has missed hearing Gaub.[59]

Gaub's next step upward came three years later when he was appointed professor of medicine at Leiden. His inaugural discourse bore the title, *On the vain expectation of prolonged life promised by chemists.*[60] He argues that neither theoretical nor practical considerations offer support to the extravagant promises of some chemists to prolong life and health by chemical means, and that the sole hope of achieving this end lies in the proper management of the non-naturals with particular attention to hygiene and diet.

At this time Gaub accomplished two very considerable feats of scholarship. In 1733 he brought out an edition of Prospero Alpini's (1533–1617) book on prognostics,[61] with a preface by Hermann Boerhaave. A few years later, in 1737, his Latin translations of Swammerdam's (1637–1680) hitherto unpublished manuscripts in Dutch were printed, together with the latter's already published works, in two huge folio volumes bearing the title, *Biblia naturae.*[62] The publication was carried out under the auspices of Hermann Boerhaave, who also provided a biographical preface. After Swammerdam's premature death Boerhaave had acquired his unpublished manuscripts and assembled them, together with already printed works, for publication.[63]

The dissertations of Gaub's students in chemistry include investigations of milk, bile and cantharides.[64] Many of Gaub's own chemical studies were collected and published under the title *Adversariorum varii argumenti* in 1771. They include analyses of the coastal waters and of the essential oils of various fruits, vegetables and nuts, and an investigation of an East Indian root, termed Jean Lopez, said to have useful properties in the treatment of diarrhea and dysentery. Gaub supplied extracts of this root to physicians in various Dutch towns who then observed its effects in practice.[65] He established relations with physicians and surgeons leaving for the Indies, urging them to look into old and well-tested local remedies.[66] Finally, he undercut a Dutch quack, Ludemann, who was peddling an antispasmodic called *luna fixa*, by revealing that the remedy consisted of flowers of zinc (zinc oxide) and establishing the proper dosage.[67] In keeping with Stahl's phlogiston theory, Gaub explained the difference between metallic zinc and zinc oxide as the result of the loss of phlogiston when the oxide was prepared, and its return when the oxide was reduced to metallic zinc.[68] Black's experiments with "fixed air", carried out from 1754 to 1757, seem to have met with some resistance on his part, as did the subsequent work of Cavendish, Priestley and Lavoisier, which took place near the end of his life.[69]

Three works are said to be the basis on which Gaub's fame rests: His previously mentioned collection of chemical studies known as the *Adversariorum*, his book on the compounding of medicines,[70] and his textbook of medicine and pathology, the *Institutiones Pathologiae Medicinalis*, in which he seeks for a middle ground in medical theory between the mechanism of Boerhaave and the psychologism of Stahl.[71]

The last named book will serve to introduce us to some recent assessments of Gaub's place in the history of medicine. It remained in use well into the nineteenth century. It is of interest that the founder of modern cellular pathology, Rudolf Virchow, used it while a medical student in Berlin in 1839.[72] Late in his life Virchow called this work the world's first textbook of general pathology and the standard until far into the nineteenth century. Boerhaave's statement with which the book began, *morbus est vita praeter naturam*, Virchow wrote, proclaimed the biological character of general pathology.[73] In Virchow's own words, the phrase meant that disease was "life under abnormal natural conditions".

In contrast to Virchow's highly favorable estimate of this work that of at least one pathologist of the present day is devastating. We search in vain, he writes, through the *Institutiones* for the solid facts that had been accumulated in the eighteenth century, through five hundred odd pages "deservedly discarded soon after the author's death" that "would not be worth the space given them here if it were not to emphasize the archaic nature of pathologic teaching at a time when Morgagni was ready to publish his encyclopedic observations on gross pathology".[74] Needless to say, Gaub can hardly be understood if general pathology is confused with pathological anatomy. The well-known German surgeon, August Bier, included an encomium of the *Institutiones* in his study of the history of the concept of inflammation,[75] and Theodor Meyer-Steineg wrote that Gaub had put the problem of the natural healing powers of the organism on a new basis in the *Institutiones* and had attempted to show in a systematic way the dependence of function on structure. Like Virchow, Meyer-Steineg regarded the *Institutiones* as the first textbook of general pathology.[76]

Gaub's two essays on psychosomatic medicine were well known in the eighteenth century, but seem to have been lost sight of, for the most part, thereafter. It was remarked above that Gaub said little that was new on this subject. Yet what he had to say is expressed clearly, forcefully, and often elegantly. Moreover, his work is informed with a considerable amount of philosophical understanding.

23

Among those who have paid tribute to him was the Viennese medical psychologist Ernst von Feuchtersleben who, about one hundred years after the publication of Gaub's first lecture on the mind-body relationship, praised his attempt to "clear up notions and principles" and his "truly philosophical views".[77] Gaub's attempt to work out a consistent mechanism of mind-body interaction in the light of current knowledge of the nervous system, his emphasis on the latter's capacity for self-arousal and on that part of it now termed the autonomic system, and, finally, his call for physicians to unite in the search for drugs capable of affecting the mind, make both of his essays still interesting today, two centuries after their composition.

Notes

INTRODUCTION

1. R. W. Gerard, for example, says that "a vital force does not move a molecule and an emotion does not discharge a neurone . . . no twisted thought without a twisted molecule." ("Biological Roots of Psychiatry", *Science*, 122: 225, 1955.)
2. See Gaub II, Note 172.
3. Eccles, John, *The Neurophysiological Basis of Mind*, Oxford, 1953, p. 272.
4. Descartes, René, *Œuvres et lettres*, Paris, 1958, p. 1157 (Lettre à Elisabeth, 28 juin 1643).
5. Goethe states this neatly in the following lines:
   Der Gott, der mir im Busen wohnt,
   Kann tief mein Innerstes erregen;
   Der über allen meinen Kräften thront,
   Er kann nach aussen nichts bewegen;
   —*Faust* I, 1566–69
6. As is often done by medical writers of the present day on psychosomatic medicine. For the problems involved see the penetrating analysis by Arthur O. Lovejoy, *The Revolt against Dualism*, La Salle, 1955.
7. Erwin Schrödinger says that we exclude the cognizing subject from the domain of nature without being rigorously systematic about it (*Mind and Matter*, Cambridge, 1958, p. 38).
8. Merleau-Ponty, Maurice, *Phenomenology of Perception*, translated by Colin Smith, London, 1962, p. 207. Smith quotes Valéry's lines from *Le cimetière marin* as the source of the phrase: *Mes repentirs, mes doutes, mes contraintes/ Sont le défaut de ton grand diamant.*
9. Gilbert Ryle calls the accepted doctrine of mind and body, "with deliberate abusiveness", the dogma of the ghost in the machine and says that it is based on a category mistake (*The Concept of Mind*, London, 1949, p. 15).
10. James, William, *Principles of Psychology*, New York 1890, 2 vols., vol. 1, p. 149. Continuing along this line, Arthur Danto argues that if machines turned out to be conscious the mind-body problem would remain as it is (*Dimensions of Mind*, ed. by Sidney Hook, New York, 1960, p. 180).
11. See Gaub II, Note 206. For further comment regarding the historical setting of the mind-body problem see Rather, L. J., "G. E. Stahl's Psychological Physiology", *Bull. Hist. Med.*, 35: pp. 42 et seq., 1961.
12. Descartes, loc. cit., also Gaub II, Note 82.

13. Hume, David, *A Treatise on Human Nature*, London, 1739, Bk. I, Pt. IV, Sec. VII, p. 269. (Reprinted from the original edition, London, 1955.)

14. See Gaub II, paragraph 26, Commentary and Notes.

15. Cabanis, Pierre Jean George, *Coup d'œil sur les révolutions et sur la réforme de la médecine*, (in) *Œuvres Philosophiques*, Presses Universitaires de France, 1956, 2 vols., vol. 2, p. 247.

16. See Gaub I, paragraph 47.

17. See Gaub I, paragraph 18.

18. See Gaub I, paragraph 19.

19. See Gaub II, paragraph 1, Commentary and Notes.

20. See Gaub I, Note 5.

21. See Gaub I, Note 66.

22. Lain-Entralgo, Pedro, *Heilkunde in geschichtlicher Entscheidung* (translated from the Spanish by Theodor Sapper), Salzburg, 1956, pp. 46–86. Spanish title is *Introducción Histórica al Estudio de la Patología Psicosomática*, Madrid, 1950. An English translation entitled *Mind and Body* was published by P. J. Kennedy & Sons, N.Y., 1956.

23. See Gaub II, 30, Commentary and Notes.

24. See Gaub II, Note 120.

25. See Gaub I, paragraph 51, Commentary and Notes.

26. Ibid.

27. Laehr, Heinrich, *Die Literatur der Psychiatrie, Neurologie und Psychologie im 18ten Jahrhundert*, Berlin, 1895.

28. *Histoire de la société royale de médecine, année 1779*, "Éloge de M. Gaubius" (anon.), Paris, 1782, pp. 118–141, p. 118. Bleuland, Jan B. *Oratio qua memoria Hieronymi Davidis Gaubii cum omnibus tum praesertim medicina studiosus commendatur*, Harderwyck, 1792, pp. 34–5.

29. Suringar, G. C. B., "Verval van het klinisch onderwijs na den dood van Boerhaave. Adrian van Roijen als hoogleeraar in de kruid- en geneeskunde. Waardering van het dynamische element in de theoretische leer van Gaubius en Frederik Winter. Pieter van Mussenbroek als hoogleeraar in de physica", *Nederlandsch Tijdschrift voor Geneeskunde*, 2e Rks., 2e Jrg., 2e Afd., Amsterdam, 1866, p. 265. A. K. Boerhaave was at that time one of Elizabeth's imperial physicians. He was also the nephew, on the maternal side, of Hermann Boerhaave.

30. Gruner, Christian Gottfried, in the preface to his translation of Gaub's *Institutiones pathologiae medicinalis*, the *Anfangsgründe der medizinischen Krankheitslehre*, Linz, 1785, p. xviii. Gruner's biographical note is based, according to his own admission, on the anonymous eulogy mentioned in Note 28.

31. Ibid., p. xviii, xix.

32. Ibid., p. xix.

33. Hahn, Johannes David, in the preface to his edition of Gaub's *Institutiones*, Leiden, 1781, p. 3. Hahn, Gaub's nephew, was called to the chair of medicine in 1775, and, according to Gruner (loc. cit., p. xii), intended to write a biography of Gaub but was prevented from doing so by his own premature death at the age of fifty-five.

34. The eulogy was read on 19 February 1782 and the opinions of the writer regarding the damage wrought by the great is therefore most interesting—"*Christophe Gaube, le plus jeune, se joignit à plusieurs de ses concitoyens; et réunis ils osèrent entreprendre de réparer les fautes de leurs Princes, en ramenant les arts et le commerce au milieu des débris dont ils étoient environnés: car l'artisan industrieux est dans les villes ce qu'est le cultivateur infatigable dans les campagnes; ce sont eux dont les grands font toujours les objets de persécution ou les instruments de leur amour-propre; et lorsque le calme est rétabli, on voit ce peuple renaissant de ces propres cendres, courir à ses travaux, et préparer de nouvelles dépouilles à de nouveaux ravisseurs*" ("Éloge de M. Gaubius", p. 119).

35. Ibid., p. 120.

36. *Encyclopædia Britannica*, 11th ed., art. Francke, August Hermann.

37. Ibid.

38. "Éloge", p. 120: "*Il existe sans doute des rapports entre les différens âges de la vie, et il est sage de prendre des précautions pour que le premier contribue au bonheur de tous les autres; mais vouloir le sacrifier entièrement à cette vue; enchaîner la mobilité de l'enfance; substituer la lenteur et la mélancolie de l'âge mûr à la saillie et aux élans des premières sensations; l'accablement à la gaîté la plus franche et la plus naïve; imposer silence à des organes qui s'essaient qui sont comme les touches d'une mémoire vraiment active; affliger enfin, tourmenter un être, qui, s'il survit, portera toujours l'empreinte du malheur et de la dureté dont on aura flétri son existence, c'est le propre de la pédanterie renforcée par l'ignorance et le fanatisme.*"

39. It was Joan Gaub who Latinized the name to Gaubius, according to the eulogist ("Éloge", p. 121) who adds—"*Les érudits affectoient alors de tenir au moins par la terminaison de leurs noms à l'ancienne Rome. On a de bonne heure secoué ce joug en France ...*". Joan Gaub survives in the medical literature as the author of two letters on anatomical problems to Frederick Ruysch written in 1695 while he was still a student and printed with replies by Ruysch, professor of anatomy at Leiden (*Johannis Gaubii epistola problematica ... ad virum clarissimum Fredericum Ruyschium ... Amstelaedami, 1724*).

40. *Specimen inaugurale medicum exhibens ideam generalem solidarum corporis humani partium ... ex auctoritate magnifici rectoris D. Joannis Ortwini Westenbergii ... pro gradu doctoratus ... submittit Hieronymus David Gaubius, Heydelb. Palatin ... 24 Augusti 1725 ... Lugduni Batavorum ... 1725.* A curious error regarding this dissertation entered the medical literature in a paper, *Die Schrift des Hieronymus*

David Gaub, De regimine mentis quod medicorum est, Inaugural-Dissertation von Karl Gutsch, Referent Prof. Dr. Martin Müller, München, 1939, which states that the *Dissertatio qua idea generalis solidarum corporis humani partium exhibetur* contains a polemic against Stahlian animism and Leibnizian pre-established harmony, although in fact there is none and their names are not mentioned. It is all the more curious since the first essay entitled *De regimine mentis,* translated in Gutsch's dissertation, does contain such a polemic.

41. "Éloge", p. 122; Gruner, p. xv.

42. *Specimen,* p. 46.

43. Ibid., p. 31.

44. Ibid., p. 9.

45. Ibid., p. 8.

46. Ibid., p. 11. The definition of Boerhaave quoted is "*corpus simplex, elementare, friabile, siccum, nec fluens, nec volatile, sed fixissimum in igne, in aqua, oleo, et aere prorsus insolubile, insipidum inodorum*".

47. Ibid., p. 13: "*... linea corpuscularis seu fibra minima solidi nostri corporis.*"

48. Gruner, p. xv. The eulogist, in praise of French methods of instruction, writes: "*... l'instruction que l'on y trouve n'est fondée que sur l'observation; c'est la science des faits que l'on vient y étudier; le professeur y est depouillé de tout appareil étranger à l'art qu'il enseigne, pour n'être que l'homme de l'expérience et de la raison; on ose l'interroger, même le contredire; en un mot, il n'a de supériorité que celle de ses connoissances, avouée par des auditeurs qui l'ont choisi librement. M. Gaubius fut très satisfait de cette espèce d'enseignement ...*" ("Éloge", p. 123).

49. "Éloge", p. 124. They were married in 1735, and had six children, five girls and a boy. All except one girl died in childhood (Suringar, p. 265).

50. Suringar, p. 264.

51. "Éloge", p. 125.

52. The eulogist's explanation of Gaub's good health during this time is instructive: "*C'est une sorte de miracle que de voir les médecins placés dans le foyer de la contagion, tout couverts, pénétrés même de ses miasmes, échapper souvent à ses coups. Ces différens virus étant du nombre de ceux qui agissent sur les nerfs, n'est-il pas vraisemblable que ces organes raffermis par le courage, et fortifiés par un bon régime, s'accoutument peu-à-peu à leurs impressions, de manière à pouvoir enfin les braver?*" ("Éloge", p. 125).

53. Suringar, p. 265.

54. "Éloge", p. 126.

55. *Oratio qua ostenditur chemiam artibus academicis jure esse inserendam, Lugduni Batavorum, 1731.* Reprinted in *Opuscula Selecta Neerlandicorum de Arte Medica,* Amsterdam, vol. 1, 1907 (with a Dutch translation), pp. 174–227.

56. *Epistolarum ab eruditis viris ad Alb. Hallerum Scriptarum*, Berne, *1773–75*, 6 vols., vol. 2, p. 101: "... *Daventriam me contuli, Praxin medicam, a qua alienissimus eram, facturus ... donec anno 1731 molestissimae praxios taedium levaret oblatum Boerhaavii favore Lectoris Chemiae in hac Academia munus ...*".

57. Ibid., vol. 3, p. 525 (letter of J. C. Ramspeck, dated 1755): "*Hora undecima summa profecto cum oblectatione audio Cel. Gaubium, Chemiam solide, clare et methodice docentem*".

58. Ibid., vol. 3, p. 336 (letter of J. F. Meckel, dated 1752): "*Bene et ordinatim utiliter res suas enunciat Gaubius, experimentis simplicibus illustrat.*"

59. Ibid., vol. 3, p. 419 (letter of de Brunn, dated 30 Sept. 1753).

60. *Oratio de vana vitae longae, a chemicis promissae, exspectatione*, Leidae, *1734*.

61. Alpini, Prospero, *De praesagienda vita et morti aegrotatium libri septem ... Editio altera Leydensis, cujus textum recensuit, passim emendavit, supplevit; citata Hippocratis loca accuravit, Hieron. Dav. Gaubius, Lugduni Batavorum ... 1733*. (In addition to a preface by Hermann Boerhaave, Gaub's edition carries a portrait of Alpini by Leander Bassanus that Gaub says he owes to the munificence of the incomparable J. B. Morgagni.)

62. Swammerdam, Jan, *Biblia naturae sive historia insectorum ... Leydae, 1737*.

63. Nordenskiöld, Erik, *The History of Biology* ... translated from the Swedish by Leonard Bucknall Eyre, New York, 1928, pp. 167–71.

64. Suringar, p. 267.

65. "Éloge", p. 132.

66. "Éloge", p. 133.

67. "Éloge", p. 134.

68. Suringar, p. 268.

69. Ibid.

70. *Libellus de methodo concinnandi formulas medicamentorum, editio altera revisa et aucta, Lugduni Batavorum, 1752*. Dedicated to Joan Gaubius and based on the *Materia medica* of Hermann Boerhaave. The first of the general rules is that the physician should prescribe nothing unless he can render a sufficient reason for its use (p. 5).

71. With reference to the *Institutiones*, the eulogist calls Gaub "plus modéré que Stahl, plus impartial que son maître." ("Éloge", p. 129).

72. "One Hundred Years of General Pathology", in *Disease, Life and Man*, Selected Essays by Rudolf Virchow, translated and with an introduction by L. J. Rather, Stanford, 1958, p. 207.

73. Ibid., p. 187.

74. Krumbhaar, E. B., *Pathology*, New York, 1937, p. 32.
75. Bier, August, "Die Entzündung", *Arch. f. klin. Chir.*, 176:407, 1933.
76. Meyer-Steineg, Theodor, "Hieronymus Dav. Gaub über die natürlichen Heilkräfte", *Arch. f. Gesch. d. Med.*, 15: 114, 1923.
77. Feuchtersleben, Ernst von, *The Principles of Medical Psychology*, translated by H. E. Lloyd, London, 1847, pp. 58, 59.

TOPICS OF THE ESSAYS AND COMMENTARY

ESSAY OF 1747

Essay of 1763

Essay of 1747

I   The Harmony of Mind and Body

1. Although the arts and sciences whose subject is man are numerous and differ greatly insofar as they deal with one or another of the aspects of man, or in different mode and measure with the same aspect, nevertheless all have a certain common bond and are bound together by a certain relationship such that they are united at some one point and cannot forego mutual support throughout.

2. Most admirable indeed is the artful union of the parts of the human body, whereby all join harmoniously together in unity in the face of the greatest differences. The faculties of the mind, too, are of the same stock and are mutually dependent, although they differ in their plan of action. Finally, the mind itself and the body, things generally held to be of entirely disparate nature, are so tightly and intimately knit when joined together in man that—if I may here speak as a chemist—they interpenetrate and dissolve in each other, so that while life flourishes, wherever there is mind there is body, and wherever body, mind. There is hardly to be found any smallest part of man in which something of mind and something of body, and in measure a mixture of both, is not to be observed.

(1) An unacknowledged debt to Cicero is evident in Gaub's opening paragraph. Cicero says, in his oration in defense of the Greek poet, Archias, that all arts pertaining to man have a certain bond in common and are bound together by a certain relationship. Gaub has clearly made use of Cicero's Latin at this point.[1]* (2a) The harmony of

* The numbers in superscript refer to the Notes.

34

the parts of the body among themselves, and of the body with the mind, are common topics in eighteenth-century medical writing. Gaub mentions the topic in his textbook, where he writes that the consensus and mutual agreement of the bodily parts constitute them into a whole that strives to preserve its integrity. When harm threatens any one part the others join their powers in resistance against the causes of disease and death.[2] (2b) When Gaub remarks ". . . if I may here speak as a chemist" we may recall that he was professor of chemistry as well as professor of medicine at the University of Leiden. Since he regards mind as something immaterial or incorporeal we may assume that "mixture" is used metaphorically. When mind or soul is thought of as a material or quasimaterial substance (as it was by the Stoics, the Methodist physicians of Greece and Rome, and certain Christian theologians such as Tertullian) the question of mixture is treated as a real one. Medical writers of Gaub's day often quote Vergil's Stoic views along these lines but mean figuratively what Vergil meant literally.[3] (2c) Note that Gaub does not equate mind with brain, for ". . . wherever there is mind there is body, and wherever body, mind".[4]

II   Effects of Body on Mind Long Recognized

3. Passing over whatever else might be brought forward, I consider that this makes one thing in particular most clearly to be understood, that the mind cannot be managed properly unless account is taken of the body to which it is joined. In turn, the management of the mind is implicit in and bound up with the proper treatment of matters pertaining to the body.

4. Thus in ancient times, in the very cradle of philosophy and medicine, the latter was ordinarily considered part of the former, and we read that the most distinguished philosophers, Pythagoras, Empedocles

and Democritus, were skilled also in the science of healing. In my opinion, this was not so much because men whose bodily powers were impaired by lack of rest and ceaseless mental activity had most need of the art of medicine, but first of all because it must have been plain to these wisest of men that health contributes more to the conservation and increase of mental vigor than does anything else, and that when the body fails it is quite likely that the mind too will suffer.

5. Nor was laborious and difficult observation indeed required to recognize something the evidence for which is as plentiful as convincing, and is set forth before men every day.

(3) In stating his belief that the proper management of the mind requires understanding and control of the body Gaub runs counter to the philosophical tradition, chiefly derived from the Stoa, calling for the treatment of mental or emotional disturbances by an appeal to the mind itself through logical reasoning, exhortation and various forms of persuasion, but taking little or no account of the body. On the other hand, however, he is well within the medical tradition exemplified by Galen's short medical treatise on the effects of the bodily temperament on the mental faculties, in which the Platonic doctrine of an incorporeal *psyché* uninfluenced by the body is rejected on the ground that this *psyché* is clearly influenced by age, diet, climate and various bodily states.[5]   (4) Gaub emphasizes the close relationship between philosophy and medicine in ancient times by pointing out that the two disciplines were frequently professed by one man (Hippocrates is traditionally credited with establishing medicine as an independent intellectual discipline).   These men, he writes, were aware of the close dependence of mind on body.   Celsus, whose *De medicina* is cited at this point by Gaub, was probably an encyclopedist rather than a practicing physician.   Gaub has borrowed Celsus' statement that the science of healing was at first held to be part of philosophy and that such celebrated

philosophers as Pythagoras, Empedocles and Democritus were expert physicians, but disagrees with his explanation of why this was so.[6] (5) It will be noted that throughout Gaub makes frequent appeals to the personal experience of his auditors.

III   The Balance of Power between Body and Mind

6. Is there any one of us, I ask, who has not himself often experienced that satiety, hunger, immoderate wakefulness, overlong repose, the drinking of wine, changes in the composition of the air, and many other things, although directly altering the bodily state alone, nevertheless at the same time strongly affect the powers of reason and understanding? Is it possible for anyone to be unaware that errors of perception, imaginative follies, and mental aberrations occur whose cure, unless accomplished with hellebore, is vainly attempted with the aid of the most exquisite apparatus of logic? Anyone who will carefully consider how greatly drunkenness, pregnancy, atrabilia and other such corporeal goads affect the behavior will further admit, I believe, that the moral no less than the rational faculties of the mind are in the power of the body, and that not every instance of intemperance, sensual indulgence, greed, inhumanity, theft, murderous rage or self-violence is always to be ascribed to the mind alone and does not sometimes issue rather from the brute body, and that the unwilling mind, it should be said, is forcibly drawn into the company of the wicked, as it were, by the body.

7. The control exercised by mind over body is indeed far more evident. Almost everyone agrees with this opinion, and someone who undertook to reaffirm it by argument might therefore seem to wish to lend light to the sun.

8. As long as the social contract of human life holds good, the power of the mind over the body is probably no greater than that of the body over the mind. Yet the mind's knowledge of the efficacy of the will and of the prompt obedience shown by a healthy body easily leads us to suppose that control has been vested in the mind and mere servitude imposed on the body. And should we not admit also that a secret pride is hidden here, inasmuch as the mind is aware that she participates in reason to a greater extent than does the body and is convinced that her right over the body is more fitting than that of the body over her? As if to command were the prerogative of reason alone! Whatever the basis of this conviction may indeed have been, it has so much weight that we seem to feel rather than believe it, nor can we doubt—much less deny— it without in a way doing ourselves violence.

9. Hence it is that those who strive to inculcate true wisdom and virtue into men's minds ought particularly to take into account, among other matters, the aids and hindrances offered by different states of the body. Reason demands with equal force that those whose calling it is to keep the human body healthy should carefully take into account the power of mind over body to aid or hinder their efforts.

(6a) The corporeal factors named here as capable of influencing the mind by way of the body are some of the traditional "non-naturals" of Galenical medicine. For a fuller discussion see commentary to §51, first lecture. (6b) Gaub probably considered it necessary to emphasize the influence of body on mind, since the influence of mind on body was a more familiar topic in his day. (6c) Later on he will argue that a person should not be held fully responsible for crimes and misdemeanors to the extent that his moral and rational faculties are in the power of the body and his actions, therefore, matters of compulsion rather than choice. (6d) In calling attention to the fact that certain kinds of mental disturbance are impervious to all appeals to the mind yet respond to agents acting on the body Gaub mentions hellebore, a powerful emetic frequently named in ancient writings as part of the treatment of mental disturbances. Details of its administration and the results are unknown. (7a) Gaub probably believed it necessary to remind his audience at this point that the body was, after all, under the control of the mind because his argument might have moved too far in the other direction for their taste. To imply that the mind, hence the person, was completely subject to the blind compulsion of the body would be uncomfortably close to religious heresy. The Augustinian strain in Christian thought emphasizes the power of the mind or soul over the body and hence the ultimate responsibility of the person for his acts. (7b) To reaffirm by argument the power of the mind over the body is like lending light to the sun because the sun is the primary source of all light and, correspondingly, our personal experience, which tells us of the efficacy of the will, is the primary source of all knowledge. (8a) Gaub ascribes as much efficacy to the mind on one hand as to the body on the other, with the difference that the mind is aware of its controlling power while the body is not. This leads the mind to overestimate its sway. To command is not always the prerogative of reason, says Gaub, clearly referring here to the irrational nature of the control exercised by the body over the mind. In his second essay, however, he cites Cicero on Stoic doctrine and apparently accepts the view expressed there that mind contains an irrational principle as well as a principle of reason. He does not attempt to reconcile these opposing views. (8b) The last sentence calls attention to the strength of our belief that we ourselves are the cause of certain corporeal activities. Gaub returns to this point several times in the course of the first essay. (9) Although both aspects of the mind-body relationship are mentioned here, it would seem that Gaub's chief wish is to state his belief that philosophers fail to accord sufficient attention to the body in their attempts to "inculcate true wisdom and virtue into men's minds", and later on (§50, First Lecture) he will quote Descartes in support of the claim that only the art of medicine can ultimately improve the moral status of mankind.

IV · Philosophers, Physicians and the Mind-Body Problem

10. Although the investigation and regulation of the faculties of the human mind appear to be the proper and sole concern of philosophers, you see that they are in some part nevertheless so little foreign to the medical forum that while someone may deny that they are proper to the physician he cannot deny that physicians have the obligation to philosophize.

11. This being the case, I shall no longer delay in disclosing to you the subject on which, in accordance with the firm rule of custom, I have chosen to speak on this occasion. I shall indeed speak of *the management of the mind as it concerns physicians*.

12. Although this has been the subject of long and bitter debate among physicians, no single opinion sits well with all. The result has been that different paths have been followed in search of cures. Have no fear that I shall trouble you with a lengthy exposition of the arguments brought forth on both sides! Not only is such a procedure quite foreign to my habits and inclinations, but also I consider it neither worthy of the dignity of this place nor of the solemnity of the day we celebrate nor, lastly, of your common attention. Therefore, avoiding partisan zeal and setting aside quarrels, I shall present, with as much brevity and artlessness as I can muster, whatever careful investigation shows to be essential to the matter. As I do so I urgently ask you to grant your favor and indulgence, which I have put to the test here at other times, toward one little versed in eloquence.

13. In order that my talk may set out from the place where its whole plan takes origin, I shall dismiss circumlocutions and call your attention to that admirable marriage which unites body and mind in man, and to its rights and duties as they are confirmed by observation. Desiring it to be peculiar to their disputations, philosophers claim for themselves the investigation of this subject, but I do not hesitate to say, with their permission, that if they see anything clearly in the darkness it would hardly be discernible but for the light borne in front by physicians.

14. No matter how often I consider the various verbal models and comparisons that are usual when this union is discussed I cannot sufficiently wonder when even men who wish to know more than the crowd frequently adopt those that depict something quite different from what each man's own mind, in the course of everyday reflection on itself and its body, ought to teach him plainly enough. In a matter of such importance, knowledge of which we have only from the sources of our deepest experience, who would not wonder?

(10) Although philosophy is not the proper field of the physician he cannot avoid philosophizing. Gaub does not refer here to the "natural philosophy" of his time, equivalent to our natural science, nor to metaphysics and ontology, but rather to ethical philosophy and psychology (the latter a philosophical discipline in the eighteenth century). The physician is chiefly concerned with man's body, as Gaub tells us elsewhere, but he cannot avoid a concern with man's mind, moral behavior and emotions, the more so since all may be involved in corporeal disease. (11) Gaub addresses his audience frequently (here for the first time) as A.O.O.H., *auditores omnis ordinis honoratissimi*, rendered here as "gentlemen". In announcing his topic he uses a slightly modified version (*De mentis regimine quod medicorum est*) of the common title of the two essays, emphasizing it with

capitals. (13) Gaub regards the "philosopher" as the weaker party in this controversy and claims that he has had to wait on the discoveries of the physician. (14) The attempts of the philosophers to solve the mind-body problem arouse his wonder, and he displays here the usual impatience of the man of science with philosophical subtleties. More important, perhaps, is his emphasis on the evidential value of inner experience, "... that which each man's mind, in the course of everyday reflection on itself and its body, ought to teach him plainly enough".[7] This is of course itself a philosophical position. He accepts inner experience as the ultimate arbiter of truth, and on this basis he will later reject Leibnizian psychophysical parallelism.

V Inadequate Solutions of the Mind-Body Problem

15. You may observe some who call the human body the home of the mind, convincing themselves and others that the mind dwells, moves freely and does everything it wishes in the body, just as each of us is accustomed to do at home. An astonishing home indeed!—on which the wisdom or folly of the mind depends, sharing dominion with its inhabitant and able to abandon its master, although he in turn cannot forsake it until he is dismissed.

16. Others consider this title too splendid, and prefer to call the body a prison or a workhouse in whose embrace the cribbed and confined mind bears a slave's yoke against its will and under duress. In truth, they take too little account of what the mind can do in the body of its own free will, nor do they consider how intensely the mind loves and anxiously watches over the body and, on the other hand, the number and extent of the aids, services and accoutrements continually heaped

up by the body that the mind would otherwise bitterly lack.

17. There are even those to whom the body seems a workshop outfitted with a complex ingenious apparatus of finished tools; they assert that the mind is at once architect and master of this factory, shaping the whole body and setting its parts in motion, and the body itself an inert mass completely devoid of all power of action, incapable of doing anything of its own free will, its instruments silent unless moved by an outside force. The mind, therefore, like a God in this machine, is the sole author of every action of the human body, even of those which we are unaware of controlling, to whom alone the construction and operation of every part is to be attributed. It may be said that men who are of this opinion must have a very remarkable sense of self-awareness to hold things dependent on their wills that others find quite beyond their control. Since this is so implausible they will merit no belief until they present the evidence from which they conclude that they voluntarily do something which occurs not only without their knowledge but even against their desires.

18. Nor does imaginative license stop here. With most unusual subtlety of spirit others have worked out a certain new form of union that is marvellously attractive to many philosophers, since it avoids the insurmountable problem of interaction between entities so different from each other. Imagine two automata, gentlemen, neither one with any power over the other, joined together with the stipulation that they have nothing in common other than a dwelling place. In each one, however, flourishes a power of action suited to its nature giving rise to a prescribed series of events, one event flowing from another in definite sequence and timing. Allow further a certain fixed and perpetual harmony between the two series of events so that those taking place at the same time in both parties coincide, one event of one series corresponding

43

and precisely answering to one of the other. With matters arranged in this fashion ought not a combination of the two appear such that the pair would seem to act on one another in reciprocal intercourse and the actions of one to be causes or effects of actions of the other, although it is precisely here that both differ? It remains, gentlemen, for you to put the mind in place of one automaton and the body in place of the other. In this way you will piece together the human being of this system, which is termed pre-established harmony. I have told you a fable whose novelty has recommended it, whose recommendation has spread it, whose spread has polished it and finally adorned it with such a pleasing look of truth that it counts among its proponents teachers of philosophy beyond the expectations of its author. I grant more than freely that if nothing more than a way for things of diverse nature to counterfeit the appearance of mutual intercourse is desired, although they rejoice in no power of reciprocal action, a more ingenious or ready to hand solution of the puzzle could not be devised. But in truth, when I see it applied to created man by men who not only seriously believe but openly profess that the harmony of the human body and mind is of just this kind, I begin indeed to wonder that in our age the play of the imagination or the power of authority still counts so heavily among philosophers that even in this matter—one more truly to be felt rather than taught— they do not hesitate to accept a fabrication so out of keeping with matters that everyone can observe in himself. I shall not just now recall how clumsily and ignorantly the mind makes use of the organs of the body in early infancy, how she gradually learns their correct use, how she becomes accustomed to the body, step by step, and the body to her. The power of acting together in orderly concert and in keeping with the laws of nature does not come to either one without effort and continual practice. This requires no proof.

I appeal, rather, to your inner awareness itself, the testimony of which, with all due restrictions, ought to be given greater consideration in this matter. Feeling pain at precisely the same instant when a part of his body is burnt with a glowing iron, can anyone be convinced that he does not suffer because he has been burnt and that he would have suffered at that very moment even if the cautery were absent? When a limb is immediately moved at the beck of the will with the force, aim, duration, and succession decreed, when, on the other hand, the will calls for repose and motion at once ceases, who can be led to believe that the body, unbidden by the mind, has done all this of its own accord? Have you not seen men whose feet or hands remain stubbornly numb and devoid of feeling? How they touch, rub and pluck at the part, as if they wanted in this way to arouse the mind to sentience? Have you observed paralytics? Exerting all powers of the will, striving as if with the whole soul to set the flaccid part in motion, they are fully persuaded that they can do this by a willed effort, as if they were still whole. Being as yet unaccustomed to their own misfortune they marvel that their limbs have cast obedience aside, and are not far from believing them no longer their own. I think that anyone who considers these things carefully and impartially will feel, more clearly than can be put into words, how weighty they are in this matter, and perhaps he will wonder, as I do, whether this offspring of ingenuity is any less suited to created man than that brought forth by the brain of a certain famous philosopher a short time ago.

(15) To call the body the home of the mind[8] in this way is to admit action of mind on body, although not necessarily that of body on mind. (16) The belief that the body is the prison house or tomb of the mind[9] (more properly of the *psychê*) can be found in Plato,[10] but Gaub probably took it from the *Tusculan Disputations* of Cicero, to judge from his

words here.[11]   Where the first comparison or model accords mind more power over body than the facts warrant, according to Gaub, the second reduces mind to the status of a prisoner. (17) The reference in this paragraph is probably to the medical system of the German physician and chemist Georg Ernst Stahl (1660–1734). His all-powerful *anima* presided, in the fashion sketched out by Gaub, over all activities of the body. An unfriendly critic might regard Stahl's *anima* as a God (or ghost) in a machine.   Gaub does him less than justice, since Stahl did attempt to draw a distinction between rational activities that were consciously willed and rational, purposeful, activities running off below the level of consciousness.   In other words he did not limit "mind" as a rational principle to "consciousness" as Gaub does at this point (Gaub is not entirely consistent throughout). Gaub asks for the evidence that we can control the organic functions—in the kidneys, for example—that take place in the absence of awareness, or control bodily activities—such as sweating or movements of the viscera—of which we may be aware but are powerless to check.   Stahl would probably have replied that this was not the point: if the functions of the body take place in accordance with a rational plan the role of the *anima* is thus defined, whether or not awareness is present.[12]   (18a) Gaub undoubtedly means G. W. Leibniz (1646–1716), and the "new form of union" is his system of pre-established harmony.   The words with which Gaub opens his description of the automata recall those of Leibniz on one occasion: "Imagine two clocks or two watches which agree perfectly with each other", and later: "Now put the mind and the body in the place of these two clocks".[13]   The problem is to explain how the perfect correspondence comes about.   Leibniz rejects the influence of one on the other (Cartesian interactionism) as physically impossible.   He also rejects the suggestion that the clocks are constantly set in adjustment (Occasionalism).   He concludes that they were so constructed in the beginning as to correspond perfectly in their movements, that is, the agreement was pre-established.[14]   Gaub, accepting the primacy of our inner experience, takes at its face value the felt interaction between mind and body—my conviction, for example, that *I* am the cause of the willed movement of my arm or leg—and appeals to the conscience or inner awareness of the members of his audience.[15]   In this light the Leibnizian solution is indeed a "fable" quite out of keeping with the data furnished by self-observation. Leibniz, however, had another problem in mind.   As he saw it, *any* physical interaction between mind and body, no matter how slight, would set the laws of motion askew. Descartes, he wrote, had believed that while mind could neither increase nor decrease the force of action of the bodily parts it could change the direction of motion by altering the flow of animal spirits in the nerves.   Had Descartes known of his "new law of nature" according to which not only total force but also direction of motion was conserved, so Leibniz wrote, he would probably have accepted the system of pre-established harmony.[16]   (18b) Gaub also opposes pre-established harmony with the argument that it would be difficult in its light to account for the long path the mind must follow in learning to use the bodily tools, although this argument has no force.   (18c) It might seem that Gaub's observations on men with paralyzed limbs could be used to contradict his own views.   David Hume did, in fact, develop the contrary argument from similar data.   Hume admits that we are aware of the power of our will to move the organs of our body, but that the means by which this is accomplished escapes us.   The mind wills a certain event and immediately thereafter a series of events "unknown to ourselves" in the nerves and muscles leads to the accomplishment of our desire.   This is solely a matter of experience, Hume claims, not a matter of knowledge.   A paralyzed man is still aware of power to move his limbs, but experience teaches him that he cannot.   Therefore there is no necessary connection between volition and bodily movement.[17]   Where Hume argues that the vain strivings of the mind to move a paralyzed limb prove that the necessary connection felt between volition and bodily movement is an illusion, Gaub argues that it proves pre-established harmony to be a fiction, presumably because it is an indication of fundamental disharmony. Like his other argument this one, too, has no force against the hypothesis of pre-established harmony, since the hypothesis is capable neither of empirical proof nor disproof. With respect to Hume, however, Gaub might with reason have said that to claim the efficacy of the will is not the same thing as to claim the unlimited efficacy of the will. In order to move a leg a man must have (at least) an intact leg. When he does move the leg he is not deceived if he takes his awareness of the efficacy of the will at its face value.[18]

VI Mind-Body Interaction and the Division of Functions: The Normal State

19. I have indeed almost been diverted from my aim by the variety of notions with which writers amuse themselves in this matter. Not to weary you with an overlong discussion, I shall dismiss all else and deal rather with that which a plain and exact survey of the human economy teaches of this mutual fellowship. Yet do not expect that I shall explain either its nature or the basis on which it rests or even, alternatively, how this subject can be approached. I confess openly and state plainly that I know and understand nothing of all these things, and moreover, I have no hope that man will ever be able to understand them. Nor shall I invent something new and seemingly more appropriate to embellish what cannot be explained. I recognize the outstanding value of analogies in teaching, but their correct use requires no little discretion. Those without deficiencies must be sought for and suitably adapted, but within measure and not beyond it. In matters of a singular and unique kind I am quite unable to see what good they can do at all, or by what right they deserve a place. Where appropriate analogies cannot be found

the absurdities of the inappropriate simply generate confusion. I consider it plain that this has happened only too often in the matter with which we are concerned.

20. Therefore, I shall faithfully set forth no more than the laws that constrain the mind and body in their fellowship, the kind and degree of their reciprocal power over each other, and the limits prescribed to the dominion and servitude of both, as they are disclosed by careful observation.

21. To begin with, I ask you to grant that everything in the human being that so takes place as to involve thought pertains to the mind. On the other hand, what there is of motion or any other feature restricted to corporeal nature is to be attributed to the body of man. Since I believe that you will grant this, I shall deal first with the kind of fellowship which is most in accord with nature and prevails when mind and body are rightly disposed, affected by neither intemperance nor weakness, and hence may be called the normal. It is very different from that seen when either one is disturbed.

22. Given a tranquil mind in a healthy body, it is evident that the mutual intercourse of the two is defined by limits such that the body communicates with the mind through some one of its parts, and in just that part in which sensation and voluntary motion are being exercised. The remaining parts are at their own disposal, managing their own affairs and yielding no obedience whatsoever to the will. For this reason there are two orders of function in man. Part of these are such that they clearly relate to both mind and body, as when something is accomplished in the body at the behest of the mind or arises in the mind as the result of changes in the bodily state. Others, however, and these of greater importance if number and need be taken into account, are purely corporeal. They are separated from the mind by so great a distance, as it

were, that they take place not only in the absence of volition and sentience but without awareness at all and even against the will. No one can be ignorant of the fact that everything termed natural or vital by physicians ought to be included here. Whether man desires it or not his heart receives and discharges blood, the arteries beat, the veins bear the blood back to the heart, the humors are circulated, food is digested and the body nourished; other things of this kind occur, their rhythm and course preserved even during sleep when the mind is quite unaware of its body, of what is taking place there, and even of itself. Nor do these activities permit of increase, decrease or interruption, even though the strongest will be brought into play. Such is the account of the second order.

23. With regard to the first that I have mentioned, however, I certainly do not wish you to suppose that the mind is entirely in power here, sitting at the helm, so to speak, in the exercise of all such activities, while the parts of the body merely obey orders. On the contrary, dominion is divided. The will presides indeed over movements of the muscles and governs them with such complete authority that they are aroused, act in turn, and desist at its beck and call. Yet does the same law hold good with regard to the senses? This is so little the case indeed that it seems necessary to say that here the body is active and the mind passive; the former commands and the latter submits. The mind can, of course, open, close, direct or avert the eyes at will by means of muscular action, but it can neither avoid seeing something that meets the eye nor avoid seeing it other than as the eye reveals it. How often is an unwilling mind tormented and troubled by hunger, thirst, and excretory needs, which we rightly number among the senses! How disconcerting it is while considering some matter for phantoms, as numerous as they are strange, to be furnished by the body even though the external senses

are at rest, how difficult it is to suppress them when they do arise, or to guard against their repeated interference!

24. This being the case, not only is mind controlled by body to the same but, I daresay, without doubt to even a greater extent than body by mind. When I consider that the nature of sensation is far more noble than that of motion, when I reflect that not all of the body can be roused to voluntary movement whereas the organs of sense are distributed almost everywhere in the body, when, lastly, I take into account the number of things that the body freely accomplishes without the command or help of the mind and, on the other hand, the few—none at all, I might almost say— that the mind accomplishes without the body, it seems almost doubtful that the former, while joined to the body, would have taken even the first step toward thought had its raw matter not come as a spur, so to speak, from the organs of sense. After thoroughly weighing and ordering these considerations with respect to one another, I find that they seem to demand rather than merely permit that I so conclude. However, enough has been said about this kind.

(19) Gaub makes it plain that he proposes to deal with the mind-body problem as a physician, not as a philosopher. He regards it as an insoluble problem in any case, since it is utterly unique and therefore incapable of being understood in any other terms. This is the meaning of his rejection of analogies.[19] (20) He will assume, therefore, that mind and body interact (we should bear in mind that he has previously called mind and body abstractions from the real unity which is man) without troubling himself about the *possibility* of such interaction. This does not mean, as will be plain in the sequel, that he will not undertake to explain the mechanism of the interaction, via the nervous system. (21a) Gaub adopts a strictly dualistic position. Everything in the human being is either corporeal or mental:

that which involves thought pertains to the mind, while motion and other features restricted to corporeal nature pertain to the body.[20] The gap between the two cannot be bridged by intermediate, quasi-material, substances, or functions. Gaub is more consistent on this point than many later writers.[21] (21b) Gaub uses the word *cogitatio* for "thought", and it is likely that he means it in the broad, Cartesian, sense of the term. Descartes states that by the word "thought" he understands everything in ourselves of which we are immediately aware, including all operations of the will, understanding, imagination and sense. This does not include whatever follows and is dependent on thought, voluntary motion, for example.[22] (22) Bodily functions are said to be of two orders:[23] those where mind as well as body are involved, and those that are purely corporeal. The latter take place in the absence of volition and awareness, or occur against the will. The first group includes sensation and willed movement of the bodily parts, both mediated by the nervous system. The second includes "everything termed natural and vital by physicians".[24] The natural and vital functions are the classical topics of physiology: circulation of the blood, digestion, respiration, excretion, etc., all of which are modifiable by the will with difficulty or not at all. (23) Gaub again emphasizes the dependence of mind on body. Even though the mind is actively in command with respect to voluntary movement, it is passive as far as sensation is concerned and must accept whatever the body offers. (24a) He regards sensation as more "noble" than motion possibly because it is more mental than corporeal (in spite of the high degree of control exercised by the body). (24b) Since the power of the mind to move the bodily parts is very limited, whereas the organs of sense to which the mind is subservient are found almost everywhere in the body and, furthermore, since the body can do much without the mind but the mind little or nothing without the body, Gaub concludes (contrary to what he has previously said) that the body is the senior partner in the alliance.

VII   Mind-Body Interaction in States
of Disturbance

25. I turn then to the other, that seen when a disturbance affects one or both of the partners.   The state of a shaken and disordered community differs from one calm and composed, and it is likewise inevitable that great turmoil will arise in man whenever some one of his parts is subjected to a violent attack, so close are the connections of the parts that form him and so united in harmony are the faculties of each part.

26. In such circumstances, therefore, we see that completely different laws and limits of mutual intercourse and of reciprocal command and obedience prevail between mind and body.   Different laws, do I say?   There are none at all!   Neither mind nor body remains within bounds.   As if utterly unconstrained by rules they strive for and exercise despotic rule over each other in turn.   You may say that the mind can then do everything to the body and the body everything to the mind, but you may equally well say that both can do nothing.   There is no function, member, or smallest part of the body that a disturbed mind cannot change and bend, as it were, to its will. Contrariwise, there is no faculty of the mind that an afflicted body cannot disturb.   When all of this occurs on both sides in such a way that neither part has self-control or can prevent the effects produced from taking place, you may more rightly call it impotence, since neither side understands how to make lawful and proper use of any of its powers to move or check.

27. Conjure up before your eyes, gentlemen—and this will not be difficult in a matter that we see illustrated in others and experience in ourselves every day— conjure up before your eyes the picture of a man whose mind is inflamed by rage or terrified by fear or excited by love or, indeed, carried away by any disturbance

whatsoever. How unlike itself is every part of his body, how devoid of control is his mind! Countenance, color, and deportment are changed, the bodily motions are altered, there are unbidden movements of the muscles, involuntary movements and uncontrollable tremors. The heart and pulses beat unnaturally, the digestion and distribution of nutriment, the circulation of the humors, the secretions and excretions—in a word, all parts of the bodily economy—are deranged. Yet the mind when undisturbed has no power over most of these activities. How greatly, then, is the dominion of the disturbed mind extended! If dominion is the proper name for a state in which that same mind has neither awareness of nor the power to check an onslaught against parts at other times most obediently following its orders!

28. This, nevertheless, is the all-powerful will to which those who have decided to concede the mind full control over every part and function of the body are wont to have recourse. A fine will indeed! Unless they place it outside of the mind altogether, they must in fact admit that the mind simultaneously desires and rejects, doing what it does not wish to do and desiring what it cannot obtain.

29. Further, we should by no means believe that it is given to the mind alone to transmit its movements and disturbances to the body. By virtue of the same mutual connection the body can no less violently assault the mind. Or is the mind of any mortal man so steadfast that he can think freely and calmly, as if he were not in torment, while plagued by the worst agonies of the gout or colic? Provided that the body be sound, anguish due to unwelcome thoughts can be routed in a variety of ways, but if it comes from a bodily affection it will not cease until the latter does, no matter what is tried.

30. When Canus Julius learned that he was soon to die, at the command of Gaius Caesar, he was

nonetheless able to remain in a peaceful state of mind, to play games and joke with his intimates and the centurion when called to his death, to comfort his grieving friends as far as the scaffold, and to philosophize tranquilly almost at the point of death itself. His zeal for philosophy had doubtless long since cast out fear of death, nor did bodily weakness at the time affect his mind. But if Caligula had been as equally able to inflict a disease on this man as to ordain his death, if he could have obstructed the philosopher's abdominal viscera with thickened humors and aroused the causes of anxiety in the body, I believe that in this way he would have triumphed over that resolute spirit. What shall I say of the effects of wine or fever? The drinking of wine affects the body rather than the mind. Fever quickens the circulation of the blood, with which a quiet mind has no commerce. Yet observe the drunkard! His mind is agitated by tumults worse than those of his body. As often as fever disturbs his brain does not a man for a time perceive, fancy, think, judge, desire, and reject far differently than when his body is sound? I pass over strokes, fits, seizures and other ailments which, upon attacking the part of the body said to be the seat of the mind, so powerfully suppress all of its faculties that they seem to be completely wiped out, the mind itself being unsure whether or not it survives. I pass over much else, since no one can be so ignorant of these matters as not to have discovered at one time or another, to his own discomfort, that he cannot always think equably, freely, and correctly, whatever the state of his body.

31. In addition, it is especially worthy of note that in whichever of the parts of man the origin of a disturbance may be, not only is it readily transmitted to the other part but is also thrown back even more vigorously to the part from which it came; as if new strength had been won the part which was first

affected is likely to be shaken again more violently than before. As a result of repeated to and fro movements the rising waves sometimes swell higher and higher and break forth at last in an agitation most difficult to control, as is common among maniacs, melancholics, and in some temperaments even in the absence of disease.

32. Hence, if all of the carefully considered facts drawn so far from reliable and everywhere available observations that I have cited here may be gathered together, I think it becomes apparent that mind and body are joined in man in such a way that as long as peaceful and nearly normal conditions obtain on both sides intercourse is cultivated to some degree at least, but that no disturbance, no really important change, can arise in one part that will not sooner or later affect the other and, what is more, be communicated to the whole man.

(25) Gaub's comparison of an uprising of the emotions to an insurrection of the populace, or some other internal disturbance of a political state, recalls Cicero's comparison of emotional disturbances to revolts against the authority of the head of a family.[25]   (26) Gaub places every part of the body under potential dominion of the mind and every function of the mind under dominion of the body.   The walls of the channels of orderly communication and action break down.   The disturbance is so great, however, that both sides are reduced to virtual impotence.   (27a) In the course of this depiction of a man in the grip of strong emotion Gaub makes the specific claim that the natural and vital functions not ordinarily subject to the mind then fall under its sway, while at the same time the mind loses its usual control over the voluntary musculature.   Both inner and outer parts are affected (in the second essay Gaub invites us to consider how much more violent and far-reaching the interior disturbances may be).   (27b) In thus extending the scope of mind-body interaction Gaub follows

medical and philosophical tradition. It is worth considering at this point how greatly Descartes deviated from the tradition in his treatment of the emotions. According to Descartes the observation of something strange or threatening sets up a movement of the animal spirits (material substances in the Cartesian scheme) in the nerves that (a) turns the neck and head, and moves the arms and legs appropriately, (b) moves the pineal gland in such a way as to incite fear or anger in the mind (not in the *brain*), and (c) in the same mechanical, reflex, fashion alters the size of the orifices of the heart and thus alters the "rarefaction of the blood". In this way a man is prepared beforehand for fight or flight.[26] The movements of the body are not primarily caused by the mind, but are rather of the nature of the reflex changes described elsewhere by Descartes.[27] Even when the body takes flight Descartes requires another movement of the pineal gland to be caused by the flow of nervous spirits in order for the mind to become aware of the flight.[28] He would not agree with Gaub that the observed disturbances of natural and vital functions indicate an extension of the mind's control over the body, but would argue that the mind had only been made aware of some shifts and changes in the bodily machinery, and that the awareness itself was mediated by a further movement of this machinery. (28) Presumably this is another reference to Stahl and his followers. What Gaub means by placing the will outside of the mind[29] is not clear, unless it is a reference to Descartes's claim that the conflicts ascribed to the clash of higher and lower parts of the mind are actually due to the clash of body with mind.[30] (29) When the body is disturbed the mind suffers along with it, Gaub points out, again emphasizing the degree to which the mind is subject to the vicissitudes of the body. (30a) The story of Canus Julius is taken from the Stoic philosopher Seneca.[31] In accounting for the courage shown by Canus Julius in the face of certain death Gaub admits a physiological factor in addition to the usual psychological or moral ones, in keeping with his aim of emphasizing what he regards as the wrongly overlooked power of body over mind. Caligula, he says, would have been able to strike fear into the victim had he been able to obstruct his viscera with thickened humors, and thus arouse the sources of anxiety in his body.[32] Gaub was a humoral pathologist like most of his contemporaries, that is, he attempted to derive the signs, symptoms and manifestations of disease, including the anatomical alterations in the organs and tissues, from pathological changes in the body fluids. The changes were those of quantity, quality and composition, the last-named including abnormal mixture and separation of the fluid components. Among the conditions he terms "diseases of coherence" in the fluids[33] are faults of excess or deficiency in coherence among the particles contained in the humors. The first is called *spissitudo* (translated above as "thickening") and the second *tenuitas*, "fineness".[34] Such derangements were thought to lead to abnormalities in position, flow and deposition of the humors. The causes of anxiety are chiefly corporeal, according to Gaub's way of thinking. Unlike hate, anger, joy, sorrow, love and the other emotions, pain and anxiety are caused *by* rather than causative *of* bodily changes. Both are classified as "disagreeable sensations arising from disease".[35] These sensations arise in the mind, and the mind is said to "sense" when it conceives ideas as a result of changes in the body.[36] The power to arouse sensations is widely distributed throughout the body, which is provided with variously equipped and appropriately disposed sensory organs for this purpose, and in this way the sensible qualities of external things are revealed to the mind. Many parts of the body are also provided with sensory organs that warn the mind of natural needs (presumably hunger, thirst and excretory needs) and when necessary compel their satisfaction.[37] Finally, the whole body is capable of giving rise in the mind to the twin warning signals of pain and anxiety. Of the two Gaub regards anxiety as the more important, and as distressing as pain.[38] Its most frequent cause is interference with respiration, which hinders the passage of blood through the lungs and thus places life in double jeopardy. Anxiety also arises when the heart cannot expel its blood or when the circulation as a whole is otherwise hindered. The underlying cause of all forms of anxiety is, he believes, a corporeal cause affecting the common sensorium so as to excite ideas in the mind that cannot be contemplated without horror and cannot be dispelled.[39] Gaub's "anxiety" has therefore little in common with the "anxiety" of modern psychiatry or theology. It is as basically corporeal in its origin as pain, and is likewise a monitor on the lookout for disturbances in the body. Gaub's conception of pain and anxiety resembles Descartes's conception of the emotions in two respects: in both cases the phenomena are regarded as basically corporeal events of which the mind subsequently becomes aware, and in both cases a definite physiological purpose is served. For a discussion of the use of artificially induced anxiety in the treatment of the insane see §96. (30b) Wine is a material substance acting on the body, yet it exerts an effect on the mind. The movement of the blood is a corporeal process, yet when it is hastened by fever the mind is at once affected. These remarks are made in order to emphasize the effects of bodily states and processes on mental states. (31) In this picturesque description of emotional reverberation or feedback the power aroused is the *enormôn*, which is introduced and discussed in the following paragraphs. (32) Gaub returns here to the point previously made in §22. The healthy mind is relatively unaware of its body. Only in states of disturbance are the barriers to mutual awareness and influence broken down.

VIII   The Power of Arousal (*Enormôn*) of the Mind

33. As often as I try to understand the rationale of this marvellous harmony, setting aside all phantasy and following nature herself, I always seem to discern a certain something both in the body and in the mind.

Whether someone wishes to call it a stimulating or arousing agent, or the *enormôn* or *hormên* of Hippocrates, or stimulus and arousal, it is all one as long as we agree about the facts. I mean just that which is the source of the impetuosity so characteristic of both emotions and bodily movements. Since they resemble each other with respect to this extraordinary power of arousal, both may be referred back to some common genus so designated. Yet it is plain that the two ought not be confused, since one has its seat in the mind and the other in the body.

34. I believe that there is indeed something in the mind that is different from the ordinary power of reflective thought, understanding, inference and judgement, different, too, from the peaceful will, yet not completely devoid of thought. When it slumbers you might think it absent entirely, so little does it then do; when it is aroused it breaks forth with a most violent impulse hardly to be contained. If you consider its origin, when it begins to erupt, you find indeed nothing more than the reflective thought with which the mind presents something to itself as good or bad, as beneficial or harmful to itself or to its body, and therefore as desireable or undesirable. When this thought is linked to the idea of a certain thing already present in the mind, the latter is immediately disturbed. Shaken by a violent impulse, as it were, it thinks and does everything in an agitated way, greatly changed from that before.

35. When a grammarian reads that Cicero called Piso an ass can he not regard this word with tranquillity and investigate and calmly set forth its origin, meaning, and variety of uses? But when he himself becomes aware that an opponent has hurled this insult at him, when the thought of the violation and affront to his good name is linked with the idea of the word, then how sudden and great is his consternation, how incessantly his thwarted mind is shaken by this furious assault!

36. What need for further examples when only too many occur every day in each man's home? The goal of my intent also forbids me to add others that would more precisely define and more copiously illustrate the matter, were my aim to treat of it here.

37. Therefore I consider one admonition sufficient. If, perchance, it seems to anyone that the source of the stormy disturbance under consideration should be sought for in the body rather than in the mind, because it becomes apparent in the body as soon as it arises, he is in fact deceived by the unbelievable speed with which disturbances of the mind are transmitted to the body. Yet no less rapidity is seen in the ordinary exercise of the senses and motion. Further, he does not properly weigh the fact that all disorders of this kind do not begin with a simple perception alone, but require further the added representation of something good or bad, seemingly in the thing presented. Thus if the most trivial material circumstance of time, place, manner of perception or the like is changed an idea that would otherwise have disturbed a man either may not disquiet him at all or may do so to a limited degree or may even have the opposite effect. Since none of these can occur without reflective thought, one can readily see that they must be ascribed to the mind rather than the body.

(33a) The discussion now turns to the sources of spontaneity in mind and body. Gaub uses various Latin and Greek terms, two of which have been left untranslated here, to indicate the matter with which he is concerned.[40] He insists here as elsewhere that he is concerned with the facts themselves and not with disputes about words, a remark that men of science were as fond of directing at philosophers in former days as they are now.[41] Neither body nor mind is a simple piece of reflex machinery waiting to be set in motion by an outside stimulus, for both possess their separate sources of spontaneous arousal. Gaub also discussed this topic in his textbook where he wrote that man was no brute machine, to accept passively injuries from without, but had a mind within.[42] (33b) The Greek terms *enormôn* and *hormên* are used by both Hippocrates and Galen. In the Hippocratic treatise on epidemic diseases the human being is divided into container, contained and moving, where "moving" is a translation of *hormônta*.[43] Galen, too, states that Hippocrates divided man into container, contained, and the moving forces.[44] Gaub repeats this division in his textbook and suggests also that the terminology of Hippocrates be retained.[45] (34) The *enormôn*, or driving force, of the mind is described here as a partly rational, appetitive, impulse, at rest a large part of the time and called into action only when the mind conceives the idea of something good or bad, desirable or undesirable. The disturbances of the mind then incited are the emotions. The *enormôn* so conceived has certain obvious relationships to the Platonic appetitive faculty, but Gaub's source is, to judge from his phraseology, Cicero's *Tusculan Disputations*. Expounding Stoic doctrine, Cicero writes that the emotions are movements of the mind called forth by an opinion (formed by the mind) of the good or bad in something that the mind represents to itself. However, these "movements" are either devoid of, contemptuous of, or disobedient to, reason[46] (see also Gaub II, 5 and commentary). (35) To use modern terminology, what Gaub means is that not the stimulus but what the mind does with it determines the subsequent course of events. He carries the argument a little further by linking the belief or opinion with thoughts already present in the mind. (36) Again an appeal is made to the personal experience of his auditors. (37a) The point is now made that the rapidity with which the disturbance becomes manifest in the body is not a sufficient reason for locating its origin there. For the disturbance does not originate in a "simple perception" but rather in the increment of good or bad that seems to be in the thing presented.[47] Its point of origin is therefore in the mind rather than in the body, since an act of judgement or reflective thought is required, and it is for this reason that the most trivial change of circumstance may completely alter a human response. The matter can be illustrated by reference to a point made by a twentieth-century psychologist: McDougall asks us to consider the case of a man who receives from a friend a telegram stating—"Your son is dead". The independence of the man's reaction to the physical stimulus can be brought out, he says, by considering the effect of omitting the initial letter of the first word. McDougall pointed to the central role of *meaning* in this episode and used it as ammunition in his attack on mechanistic psychology. There are, of course, ways in which "meaning" (of a kind) can be interpreted mechanistically.[48] (37b) The dispute about the status of the judgement of the good or ill present in the thing or situation confronted is too complicated to be dealt with exhaustively here, but some remarks must be made. The early Stoics, according to A. E. Taylor, committed the "intellectualistic" error of identifying emotions with judgements, so that of the four primary emotions pleasure and pain were identified with the belief that one is in present possession of a good or evil, and hope and fear with the belief that good or evil are impending. One of the most important changes made by the later Stoic, Posidonius, was to return to the Pythagorean-Socratic doctrine that the emotions pertain to the irrational part of the soul.[49] Posidonius, according to the testimony of Galen, argued that the emotions were neither false judgements nor their consequences, and were thus not functions or manifestations of the rational part of the soul.[50] Some of the ambiguities in the Cartesian conception of the emotions are due to Descartes's attempt to fuse his physiological "reflex" theory with the traditional Stoic view that the emotions are the result of a judgement of value. The reflex theory of the emotions, as worked out by Descartes, is the basis of modern behavioristic psychology, since it displaces the "soul" or "mind" to the position of a mere observer, or nearly so. Descartes ignored the problem of "judgement", which is crucial to any theory of the emotions, although he could have dealt with it by regarding the brain as a calculating machine in which the sense data were assembled and interpreted. The long history of this question is not closed.[51]

IX   The Corporeal *Enormôn* and the Nervous System

38. The body, too, has an *enormôn* or agent of arousal that shares its corporeal nature and therefore lies outside of the mind and is the most outstanding feature of the living body, perhaps deserving of the name life itself. It is the principle of motion of all parts of the body, from which all of those movements spontaneously carried out by the body in the absence of awareness of the mind are derived; it seems also to cause the residual twitching seen in parts of living creatures cut off or torn away. Through its mediation and aid the organs of sense and motion quicken the mutual intercourse of mind and body. Finally, together with its companion, which I have just now located in the mind, it storms through every part of a disturbed man with unchecked fury.

39. If we carefully consider what can be observed in the body in both health and disease, it appears plausible that what I call the agent of arousal has its seat in that part of the body constituted by the origins and processes of the nerves. It would seem that this part might without impropriety be termed the neural man. It is distributed throughout the entire body and so intermingled with each of its parts that if separated from these parts it could present a simulacrum or skeletal image of a man. Furthermore, this structure of nerves is no less animated from within by its motive power than it itself stirs up the rest of the body's inert mass throughout which it extends. In this sense it represents a kind of man within a man.

40. The different plan of the movements carried out requires indeed that some division be made. We cannot now discuss whether there are actually two distinct systems, whether they are of double origin but become unified in the course of development, whether they supply different territories, or, finally, whether all distinctions depend solely on differences in the principle and laws of motion.

41. It is certain that in the healthy state the part of the neural man superintending the senses and voluntary movements has a very close relationship to the mind. Whatever it does is done with the knowledge, understanding, or even at the command of the mind. The mind knows when it is affected, and, contrariwise, when the mind commands it promptly obeys. An agent of arousal, an *enormôn*, transmitting its changes of state through the organs of sense to the mind, is therefore present in this part, and so also the mind's choice is evident in the production of movements. This part can therefore be regarded as a kind of intermediary through which the mind and the organs of the body communicate.

42. As I remarked above the other part, to which the natural and vital functions are committed, is itself constrained solely by its own laws. These are in no way derived from the mind, since it is its own master and the will has no direct power to excite, alter or prevent its movements. Hence the principle of arousal by which this part is ruled is likewise independent and quite different from that of its counterpart, since it lies beyond the power of the mind and has nothing in common with the latter.

43. Yet who would venture to hold that these two principles of motion disclosed in the body are as different in nature as they are different in relation to the mind? Vouched for by evidence that cannot be doubted, it is certain that their difference—if such be allowed—does not in any way prevent them from

acting together in mutual agreement or from transferring their states to one another. That pain frequently causes fever is surely clear enough proof that strongly affected sense organs disturb the motive power supervising the circulation of the humors. To give only one example, the state of confusion so often arising from fever teaches us that this powerful impetus is not brought to bear against the body without in turn affecting that principle animating the organs of sense.

(38a) In accord with his mind-body dualism Gaub has separated the driving force, or source of spontaneity, of the body from that of the mind. The *enormôn* of the body is itself corporeal. It is the principle of motion and source of spontaneous movement in bodily parts that have been cut away from the main mass. Elsewhere he states that the residual motions seen in excised parts of living bodies make it plain that there are corporeal motive forces that are quite independent of the mind.[52] The same observation, it may be remarked in passing, was used by La Mettrie and others to dispose of mind altogether. (38b) Gaub's more famous contemporary, Albrecht von Haller, had already shown that muscle tissues were the contractile elements of the animal body, and had designated the contractile response as *irritabilitas*, irritability. Gaub is concerned here with a broader problem, that of the corporeal source of spontaneous movement. His ideas are rather reminiscent of those of Francis Glisson (1597–1677), who has been called the true father of the doctrine of irritability.[53] Glissonian irritability is at once more broadly conceived and less well defined than Hallerian, and is perhaps more along the lines indicated by Gaub: a local principle of life. (39) The corporeal power of arousal, the *enormôn* of the body, is now located in the nervous system, which is called here a skeletal image and simulacrum of a man because its components are so widely and uniformly distributed throughout the body. The nervous system is the source of motion in the solid parts of the body just as the heart is the source of motion of the fluid parts. Yet the nervous system is itself animated from within by a motive power.[54] Gaub neither means to postulate a third *enormôn* here nor to assign the mind the role of the animator of the nervous system, as the following paragraphs show. What he means is that the nervous system itself, including its own source of arousal, is the corporeal *enormôn*, in contrast to the incorporeal *enormôn* of the mind. (40) He now distinguishes two related sources of spontaneous activity within the nervous system. He has stated above (§22) that bodily functions are of two kinds, (a) those of which we are aware or can voluntarily control (sensation and voluntary motion), and (b) those of which we are unaware or cannot control (circulation, respiration, digestion, excretion and the other natural and vital functions). Both are mediated by the corporeal *enormôn*, that is, the nervous system. He now raises several questions. Are there two distinct nervous systems[55] corresponding to the two sets of functions? Are there two systems with separate origins which later become unified? Do they supply different parts of the body? Or do all distinctions depend solely on differences in the laws governing the systems and their principles of motion? (41) That part of the nervous system—called here figuratively the "neural man"—concerned with the mediation of sensation and voluntary movement is more closely related to the mind than the other part (governing the natural and vital functions). It is, in fact, the medium through which mind and body communicate.[56] Gaub is consistent in his mind-body dualism and does not equate the mind with the brain or with the nervous system as a whole. The mind acts *through* the nervous system, through a part of it at least, and contrariwise the nervous system conveys information about the body to the mind. (42) The natural and vital functions, on the other hand, are controlled by a part of the nervous system that is not only almost independent of the mind but provided as well with an *enormôn* relatively independent of the *enormôn* of the part of the nervous system mediating sensation and voluntary movement. The will has no power to excite, alter or prevent movements of the bodily organs presided over by this element. (43) Gaub does seem to have given us two corporeal *enormônta* or centers of arousal in the place of one, but his remarks can be interpreted along the following lines. He believes that the mind is by nature simple and indivisible, whereas the body is complex and multipartite. The nervous system as a whole is the driving mechanism of the body (as well as the source of information to the mind about the body). However, there is no inconsistency involved in breaking down this complex mechanism into component and semi-independent parts. As he tells us in this paragraph, the two principles of motion[57] are related to each other. They may act together and interchange states, as when pain (a sensation, mediated by the first system) causes fever (a circulatory disturbance, Gaub believes, involving the second system) or when fever affects the quality of sensation. What he has done here is to sketch in outline the voluntary and involuntary (sympathetic, autonomic, or vegetative) nervous systems of modern physiology. His conception of the autonomic or involuntary nervous system is based on clinical observation and functional analysis rather than on anatomical investigation. It is evident from the questions raised in §40 that the topic was under discussion, and he does not indicate that his ideas are in any way novel. We may assume that he was familiar with Jaques-Benigne Winslow's anatomical description of the sympathetic nervous system.[58]

X   The Mechanism of Interaction of Mind and Body in Emotional Disturbances

44. If anyone carefully considers each and compares all of these matters with one another, it will not be difficult for him to see just how it comes about that the limits drawn by nature with regard to the fixed concord of mind and body and to their powers of mutual intercourse, which I have discussed above, are so far

overstepped when an outstanding disturbance takes place on either side. The *enormôn* of the mind previously mentioned doubtless has the closest relationship to that part of the principle of bodily arousal which controls the animal functions. There is also an open accord between this and the other part of the principle which controls the remaining bodily functions. Therefore, is it not inevitable that as soon as a sufficiently severe disturbance arises in the mind not only will a violent impulse at once be transmitted to the organs of sense and voluntary motion, but also that the whole body will be affected in turn by its force or persistence? The same outcome is to be expected when disturbances of sufficient severity arise in the body. For in whichever of its systems the first waves arise, it can hardly be otherwise than that when they are massive or persistent they will be transmitted to the other parts of the body and, in the end, to the mind itself.

45. I believe that I have said more than enough about these two modes of intercourse between mind and body. It was necessary to set forth the matter in detail, since the crux of the regimen of which I shall speak is found to lie here. What remains to be said can be presented in a few words, and you need not be alarmed by the thought that my time has almost run out.

(44) Bearing in mind that it is not Gaub's aim to show how the problem of the *possibility* (the philosophical problem) of mind-body interaction can be solved we can see how he envisages the mechanism of that interaction. The *enormôn* of the mind first acts on the part of the nervous system (the corporeal *enormôn*) controlling sensation and voluntary movement.[59] This part of the corporeal *enormôn* affects, in one way or another, the part which governs the natural and vital functions of the body. In other words, any felt emotional disturbance of sufficient degree will first affect voluntary motion and sensation and then the circulation, respiration, digestion, excretion and so forth. The same

series of events will play off in reverse order if the initial source of the disturbance is in the body rather than the mind. (45) The two modes of intercourse are direct and indirect, respectively, the direct effect on sensation and voluntary motion and the indirect effect on the natural and vital functions.

XI   The Physician's Duty is to Care for the Whole Man; Mind and Body are Abstractions

46. All of you know that we apply the term physician to those who properly supervise man's health, maintaining the good and correcting the bad. If health is the aim of the art of medicine, it clearly follows that whatever can be done to retrieve it when it is lost or to support it when it is present pertains to medicine, inasmuch as the task of medicine is to understand rightly the natural safeguards of health, whatever they may be, and to apply each one of them wisely in accordance with the aim of the art.

47. Although this healing aspect of medicine properly looks toward the human body only, rather than the whole man, it has reference to a body closely united to a mind and, by virtue of their union, almost continuously acting on its companion as well as being affected itself in turn.   In his thoughts, to be sure, the physician can abstract body from mind and consider it separately in order to be less confused in the marshalling of ideas.   Yet in the actual practice of his art, where he has to do with man as he is, should the physician devote all of his efforts to the body alone, and take no account of the mind, his curative endeavors will pretty often be less than happy and his purpose either wholly missed or part of what pertains to it neglected.   For there is a great power of action in the harmony and agreement mediating between these two parts of man, permitting them not only to act on each other but even to

interchange various states. Hence the reason why a sound body becomes ill, or an ailing body recovers, very often lies in the mind. Contrariwise, the body can frequently both beget mental illnesses and heal its offspring.

48. This being so I think it more than clear that the physician, especially when engaged in his work, should not completely overlook the mind but should rather devote some part of his care to it and see whether it can be helped by changing the body, or again whether the cause or cure of the disease troubling the body is perchance to be found in the mind. Hence it remains for me to point out just what is included among the duties of the physician in the care of the mind.

49. As I survey in thought the immense field of the practice of medicine I seem to discern two times and occasions in which it, more than any other art whatsoever, is required to give care and guidance to the mind. I believe, therefore, that the entire subject can conveniently be covered under the same number of headings. In one set of circumstances the mind is distressed because of a deranged bodily state or, though ailing on its own account, can be healed by remedies acting on the body. In the other the mind causes the bodily disease, or the disease can be suppressed by remedies acting on the mind. In the one case mind is ruled by body, in the other body by mind. I had intended to discuss both at this time, but I perceive that the wealth of material and the interest of the subject have kept me to preliminaries longer than is fitting. Changing my plan, therefore, I shall not discuss the latter aspect of this regimen, even though it is the more important. So many and so weighty are the matters involved that they would require a longer discussion than I would wish to force on you or than you could patiently hear. I shall therefore discuss only the former aspect, where the physician is to have regard for the mind while caring for the body,

since what is here of importance can be summed up briefly.

(46) Gaub admits that the physician's first concern is with the health of the body. (47) But he wants it understood that the body, as such, is an abstraction from the whole man made for the convenience of the physician.[60] In practice the physician must deal with man as he is,[61] and man is an indissoluble compound of body and mind as long as he lives. The requirement that the physician concern himself with the mental condition of his patients, in particular with respect to emotional disturbances, can also be found in Gaub's textbook. He writes that although medicine deals primarily with diseases due to bodily derangements, these diseases may have causes lying in the mind. Furthermore, all disturbances of the human functions potentially lie within the province of medicine, since hidden bodily disease may be exerting great influence in patients whose minds alone seem involved.[62] Later on in this essay (§82, 83, 90) he will state that the bodily cause of an ailment of the mind may be extremely difficult to detect, hence the physician must investigate his patients with the greatest care before ruling such causes out of court. This is one of Gaub's most important points, to which he returns again and again. (48) The emphasis here is on practice rather than theory. It is especially in the practice of his art that the physician must pay attention to the mind, in particular to the emotional disturbances of his patient. (49a) That Gaub has a practical rather than a theoretical goal before his eyes is made quite plain in this paragraph. Depending on therapeutic needs of the moment the physician may find it expedient to treat his patient either as a physical organism or as a person. Whether a mental illness or emotional disturbance is caused by a bodily derangement or not, if it can more readily and successfully be treated by treating the body the physician should take advantage of the fact. Conversely, if treatment directed at the mind will benefit a patient with a bodily ailment it is the business of

the physician to apply this treatment, whether or not the bodily ailment has causes lying in the mind. In the first case drugs, diet and other remedies acting directly on the body are called for, in the second case the patient is to be treated by moral exhortation, persuasion, advice, induced emotions (a topic covered in the second essay) and, where possible, amelioration of his social and personal life. Ultimate causes are not the physician's concern, Gaub writes in his textbook. His "causes" must be related to "remedies". They are such that the disease in question appears when the cause is present, persists only so long as the cause is active, changes when the cause changes and disappears when the cause ceases to act.[63] (49b) The twofold character of the physician's role follows from the fact that in one set of circumstances mind is ruled by body, in the other body by mind. Gaub's statement that for lack of time he will discuss the former only is probably rhetorical. It is more likely that he believed his audience to be sufficiently well acquainted with the effects of mind on body and wished to emphasize the other aspect of the relationship. The last sentence is slightly ambiguous but means that he will discuss the various ways in which treatment directed at the body can benefit the mind.

XII   A Defense of the Physician's Concern with the Body in Caring for the Mind

50. I certainly do not deny that at first sight it may appear, not without reason, that a physician who undertakes to deal with this subject is wielding his scythe in a stranger's field and, as if he had insufficient occupation in his own art, rashly claiming as his own that which properly belongs to the philosopher. After having carefully considered the matter, if someone still does not hesitate to raise this objection I would have him know that it should be regarded as care of the body rather than of the mind, although

indeed such that the mind, too, is helped by the same exertions when the body's parts are altered under the guidance of the physician. For this reason I have called it the management of the mind by means of the body. If this excuse seems less than acceptable, then let us act, physicians! Let us withdraw our hands from ailments of the mind! Let the philosophers have each and every one of them without exception! As long as the number of bodily ailments is so great our doorways will not be lifeless. Let the same law that they impose on us apply to them in turn, however, so that they do not presume to plow with our calves when perchance they profit too little with their own. If the give and take of this bargain does not displease them more quickly than it does us, I am deceived! Rather let the philosophers, in friendly agreement, yield to physicians the kind of mental care resting on management of the body, to the end that the nobler part of man may be the more happily perfected by the common zeal of both. Yet what need is there to extort by force something that Descartes, the most ingenious philosopher of his age, not only yielded to physicians but granted as proper, without any entreaty on their part? He states quite frankly that "the mind depends on the temperament and state of the bodily organs to such a degree that if any way can be discovered to make men wiser and more talented than they have heretofore been we must suppose that it should be looked for in the art of medicine".

51. And so if a sound mind is present in a sound body the physician will, by keeping the body healthy and whole with the aid of salutary hygienic precepts, see to it that the integrity of the mind is maintained. Since minor bodily changes caused by errors in mode of life often present very great hindrances to the mind, and since it cannot always function with the same readiness regardless of whether the body is situated in a moist or dry climate, or too much or too little food is

eaten or water or wine drunk, or sleep is excessive or insufficient, the physician's task is to set forth the choice, order and manner of climate, food, exercise, and the other so-called non-naturals, that each particular person must observe so that the mind may enjoy enduring strength and unbroken clarity.

52. Although men endowed with enough strength of mind and body to do everything freely and without harm are found, who are in consequence not bound by rules and do not need the physician—except to advise some of them that it is too late to be sorry and that they have expected too much from their powers—they are nevertheless very few among the many. On the other hand, particularly among men devoted to the cultivation of mind rather than body we see far more who are endowed with feebler bodies and are obliged to cherish their health carefully else they will find themselves unable to engage in long and demanding intellectual activity without great inconvenience.

53. Moreover, there is sometimes a need for intense and continuous activity of the mind beyond its power to accomplish without harm. Unless the body is then given medical attention it may indeed be rendered sluggish by fatigue or broken by pain and desert the mind in the middle of the task.

54. If by any chance it still appears to anyone that such matters are not of sufficient importance to require the aid of a physician (on the grounds that vigor of the mind often returns of itself as a result of nothing more than the rest and restraint demanded by weariness and indisposition) it is necessary to remind him also that this is indeed not always the outcome, for instances are not lacking of men who have in the end been so weakened by prolonged mental activity that, their acuity quite blunted by neglect of the body, they have fallen into folly and even feeble-mindedness.

55. The activities of the human mind are in general such that almost all of them require at least some aid

from the body, the latter supplying either the stuff of thought or the instruments with which the mind accomplishes what it wishes. Although some indeed may hold that part of these activities are carried out with no assistance from the body, it is nevertheless quite certain that both these and all others can to a very great extent be prevented from taking place rapidly and properly as a result of bodily interference. It follows therefore that all of them will be more freely and fully accomplished to the extent that the state of all bodily parts exactly meets the conditions of best health.

56. Unless we wish to hold that the unparalleled correspondence of the parts of the body under the command of the mind has happened without any reason, that the divine workmanship which we admire here is more ornamental than useful, and that any arrangement of the parts used by the mind would have been equally appropriate, we must of necessity admit that the kinds of activity carried out by the mind with the aid of the bodily organs are not so completely in its power that their different disposal would have neither greatly helped nor hindered.

57. The rationale of the perceptions coming to the mind from the body is in no way different. The various states of the organs ought in fact to have even more importance here, since it is most likely that in this interchange the mind is passive rather than active. Which one of us has not found the same thing to seem very different in one way or another according as the organ of sense that it affects is differently disposed at various times? What discrepancies in matters of taste are brought forth by age or illness! The tender palate of the child was once disgusted by something that often becomes quite agreeable to the grown man. It is an everyday observation of physicians that a drink, which had shortly before been agreeable to a feverish man, seems distasteful after the fever has departed— only to become agreeable once again when the fever

returns. To anyone capable of observing himself, there is no one of the external senses that fails to offer numerous and convincing instances of this fact. The so-called internal senses are of the same order, as is made plain by dreams and madness to mention nothing else. It is of great importance to recall here that the bodily organs have enough power over the mind to be capable at times even of deceiving the understanding by the transmission of perceptions of things that the mind knows very well are absent and cannot possibly be perceived. Men born with and accustomed to the use of sound bodies who have had the misfortune later to lose some member often learn this to their own great discomfort. Even though they are only too well aware of their loss the most unshakeable conviction of this fact does not prevent them from repeatedly seeming to feel pain in the selfsame part of the body that they know to be missing, and they attest to the pain as heatedly and unequivocally as if the part had never been lost. What a deception! To locate its source in the mind does not have the look of truth, therefore it may fittingly be referred to the body.

58. Lastly, even if the mind does have the power to carry out certain activities in such a way that they are wholly confined within and have no bodily component, it is nevertheless certain that changes in the state of the body to some extent affect these activities too. I shall pass over the great difficulty of understanding how a reasonable and continuous flow of thought can be maintained if the external senses, the memory and the imagination, the greater part of which, to say the least, the body can claim as its own, do not continually supply images. Suffice it to say that mind and body are always watchfully in touch, and at every moment one is being acted on by the other. You will find very few men, therefore, who can so withdraw the mind from the body that it can carry on its thoughts alone and in its own chamber, so to speak, unaffected by the many

changing conditions of the mutual relationship. Repeated interruptions on the part of the body disturb and prevent most of us from holding steadily to the contemplation of any one subject. All of us can readily observe how we are more or less affected at different times in accordance with our varying use of the non-naturals: more when the bodily parts are upset and aroused to disorderly activity by an irregular regimen, and least when the whole bodily economy has been adapted to the measure of good health by a proper mode of life.

59. If anyone will carefully consider these matters he will no longer remain in doubt, I believe, that when the physician through his art puts the body in an optimum state of health by the same token he greatly helps the mind, at once furthering and perfecting all of its activities.

60. Although this aspect of the physician's task is rarely taken into account, that it should not be relegated to the last place or slighted altogether is most plain from the fact that it concerns not only man's power of understanding—with which many can readily dispense in the absence of great inconvenience to themselves or detriment to the community—but first and foremost his character. No less wise than true is the statement of one of the ancient philosophers that "since the mind flourishes when health prevails it is fitting that those who are well aware of this make provision for the latter: indeed, where the state of the body languishes neither is the mind ready for the practice of what is best". Among those who teach moral precepts there is surely no one who does not moreover know that the human virtues and vices arise from the emotions or, even if they do arise elsewhere, are very much influenced by them. Since these emotions themselves are stirred up by that power of arousal previously attributed to the mind, and since the agreement of this power with the principle of bodily

motion is as complete as it is continuous, is there any doubt but that the physician who renders the *enormôn* of the body more lively and active by the appropriate use of the non-naturals, or, when overactive, calmer and more subdued, is, although he treat the body only, not entirely devoid of power to control at the same time those impulses of the mind that are the sources of so many goods or evils? Is there any one of you who does not know that the venereal appetite may be aroused or checked by food and drink, by various atmospheric conditions prevailing at different times of the year, or even by odors alone? Who is unaware of the marvellous power of wine to summon, suppress or abolish the emotions? Trustworthy observations show that the dispositions of men and beasts become savage and cruel from the use of bloody foods, whereas they are made gentle by those brought forth by the earth. Hence it is likely that men who abound with wealth and indulge their palates and bellies with whatever excess can contrive, who taint their offspring from early childhood on with the same intemperance, in this way often put great obstacles in the way of virtue, both for themselves and their children, and sharpen the spurs of vice, which they are the less able to resist the more it is nourished by intemperance and continually furnished new food by the lustful body.

61. Should we not therefore follow our forebears, wise men like Plato, Pythagoras and other ancient philosophers, who devoted part of their teaching to the regulation of the diet in order to help the mind attain virtue by caring for the body? The early lawgivers of the people saw the matter in the same light, since they too did not forget to prescribe for them dietary rules, especially those to be followed in the raising of children, and to prohibit certain foods and drinks. Although the many reasons for making such decrees were not the same for all of these men, in my opinion doubtless one of the many was that, having made the

bodies of their citizens resistant to all intemperance by a right way of life, they would at the same time keep their minds less hampered in the flight from vice and the exercise of virtue. It is surely for no other reason that Plato limits the use of wine in his commonwealth with laws so stringent that he seems almost to want to restrict it to the ill. After a thorough discussion of the subject he does not hesitate to conclude as follows: "I much more approve of Carthaginian law than of the custom of the Cretans and Lacedaemonians, however, since water is drunk during the entire stay in camp and no one dares to touch wine. In the city I would not permit wine to slaves, to magistrates during their terms of office, to prefects and judges engaged in official duties, or indeed to anyone about to consider a matter of importance. It is plain, too, that no one should drink during the day except in consequence of illness or bodily exertion, nor should a man and woman by night when they wish to have children. In addition, many other circumstances could be mentioned in which men of upright mind and principle ought not drink wine."

(50a) The treatment of mental and emotional disorders is clearly within the province of the physician when the measures applied affect the body directly and the mind only indirectly. We recall that for Gaub direct treatment of the mind includes advice, exhortation, admonition and therapeutic induction of emotion—the application of meaningful words and situations (the latter to induce emotions) in contrast to drugs and surgery. The novelty of Gaub's position, in his own eyes, lies in his proposal to expand the use of available agents acting on the body and to seek out new ones. (50b) Gaub fears the protest of the philosopher, meaning of course the moral philosopher. One would assume that much of the moral exhortation customary in dealing with emotional reactions in his time came from the mouths of divines,[64] but Gaub's words suggest that there were practicing "philosophers" who not only treated mental disturbances with moral exhortation and so forth but at times used drugs and physical agents when these means failed.[65] To the modern reader this has overtones of a dispute between physicians and clinical psychologists over the boundaries of their domains. (50c) Gaub cites a passage from a Latin version of Descartes's *Discourse on Method* at this point.[66] Descartes goes on to say that we could free ourselves from a large number of ailments of the body and mind, as well as from the ills and weakness of old age, if we knew the causes of these conditions and were acquainted with the remedies provided by nature. He then calls on men of good sense to engage in the search for the means to this end and to publish the results of their experiments so that new workers can begin where the older leave off. This is Gaub's wish as well, and in §97 he calls on all physicians to join their efforts in the prosecution of the task. (51a) It would seem from this paragraph alone that Gaub in making use of Juvenal's phrase "a sound mind in a sound body" meant to imply that a sound mind could only be present in a sound body.[67] This is evidently not his meaning, however, since in §83 he presents the case of a dull-witted youth transformed into a moral philosopher by fever and approaching death. (51b) In his textbook Gaub states that the field of the physician's activities may be divided into hygiene and medicine. Hygiene includes (a) physiology: the study of the economy of the human body, including the nature of and the factors determining life and health, (b) physiological semeiotics: the study of the signs of different grades and states of health, and (c) dietetics: the study of the measures for promoting life and health. Medicine includes the counterparts of these three, (a) pathology: the study of the nature, causes and effects of disease, (b) pathological semeiotics: the study of the signs and symptoms of disease, and (c) therapy: the study of the measures useful in the treatment of disease.[68] (51c) Gaub says that the "non-naturals" are so called because they are neither in accord with nature (*secundum naturam*) or against

nature (*praeter naturam*). They are general factors determining disease and health, in themselves neither helpful nor
harmful but becoming so when they are used or abused,
respectively.[69]   He assigns all causes of disease to three
categories, (1) the body, (2) the mind, (3) the externals.[70]
The conception of the "non-naturals" is explicitly set forth
by Galen, although he does not use the term.[71]   The non-
naturals continued to be discussed by physicians down
through the eighteenth century.   Gaub's teacher, Hermann
Boerhaave, preferred a somewhat different classification,
which may be of interest here.   He distinguished proximate,
predisposing and occasional causes of disease.   Proximate
causes invariably produced the disease in question if present,
predisposing causes were continuously acting factors
favoring a given disease, and occasional causes were those
capable of exciting the predisposing causes.   He divided
the occasional causes into four classes: (1) things taken into
the body, (2) things retained in the body, (3) things applied
to the external surface of the body, (4) actions, including the
emotions,[72] and remarked that they could less conveniently
be divided into the six non-naturals: (1) air, (2) food and
drink, (3) motion and rest, (4) emotions or affections of the
mind, (5) retentions and excretions, (6) sleeping and
waking.[73]   (52) The amount of care for the body required
to maintain the mind in good condition is seen to vary from
person to person.   The differences in constitution met with
among men were perhaps more strongly emphasized in
traditional Galenical medicine than in modern medicine,
where the disease entity plays a much more important role.
Gaub was nevertheless dissatisfied with the amount of
medical attention devoted to these differences (see §77, 78).
   (53) The intense and continuous activity of the mind
referred to here is not merely the activity of abstract thought
(see commentary to §21).   (54) Eighteenth-century medical writers frequently describe cases of insanity or feeble-
mindedness resulting from overstraining the mind.   The
topic is also discussed in Gaub's textbook under the heading of
"immoderate use of the mind".   We can scarcely conceive

of any act of the mind, he writes, that does not involve the body in one way or another. When severe and prolonged thought is required the organ of the mind (the brain) is alternately stimulated, relaxed, tensed or otherwise moved. The nervous system is involved, whether through flow of the so-called animal spirits in the nerves or in some other way. The end result may be sleeplessness, progressive loss of nervous strength, confusion and even fatuity.[74] (55) The body supplies the mind with the stuff of thought[75] or the instruments with which it accomplishes its desires. This means that the mind works with information derived from the bodily senses and that it makes use of the brain and the other parts of the body to carry out its aims. In the passage from his textbook cited above Gaub implies that thought never occurs in the absence of a corporeal change, while here he says that even if it does it is subject to bodily interference. (56) The point here is that if the mind were capable of operating independently of corporeal limitations we would be hard put to account for the precise adaptations of the body to the activities of the mind and the limitation of the power of will to those activities made possible by the arrangement of the parts of the body. When Gaub rejects the notion that "any arrangement of the parts used by the mind would have been equally appropriate" he does so, implicitly at least, under the influence of the principle of sufficient reason. Gaub's words imply a kind of pre-established harmony. (57) The mind's power of awareness is dependent on the organs of sense, and these in turn on the varying states of the body in health and disease. The internal senses, so called,[76] referred to here evidently are the "interior senses", whose history has been traced by H. A. Wolfson. In Latin philosophical texts the term refers to the three spiritual as opposed to the five corporeal senses: imagination, cogitation and memory. The same meaning is found in Arabic and Hebrew texts. The three interior senses are located in the anterior, middle and posterior hollows of the brain.[77] In the case of the "phantom limb" Gaub assigns the responsibility for the

deception to the body because the mind knows that the limb
is actually missing.   Rather than as a deception of the mind
by the body the phantom limb might seem to represent a
failure of the mind to resolve the conflicting evidence of the
senses, but this too is not an altogether satisfactory way of
explaining the matter, as Merleau-Ponty has shown.[78]
(58) Gaub recapitulates the argument of §55, pointing out
that the mind has maximum freedom when the non-naturals
are put to optimal use.   (60a) Gaub regards this neglected
part of the physician's role as all the more important in view
of the fact that the moral behavior or character[79] of man,
rather than his intelligence, is at stake.   The community
or the individual can dispense with the one more easily than
the other, he claims.   (60b) Gaub attributes the quotation
here to a letter by Democritus or "some other person"
included in the Hippocratic works.   This letter is regarded
as spurious by modern philologists.[80]   It states that all
men should have some knowledge of the art of medicine.
Philosophy is the sister of medicine; she delivers the mind
from disturbances of the emotions, while medicine relieves
the body from disease.   The letter then continues with the
passage quoted by Gaub.[81]   (60c) The emotions are
stirred up by the driving power of the mind, and Gaub has
previously described the close bond between the driving
powers of the mind and body.   It is therefore within the
physician's power to control indirectly the *enormôn* of the
mind by arousing or subduing, as need be, the *enormôn* of
the body.   This is to be done by the appropriate use of the
non-naturals, that is, by prescribing a regime fitted to the
needs of the individual concerned.   (60d) Gaub now shifts
to a discussion of the effects of some of the non-naturals.
(61) The closing sentences of the last paragraph and the
opening sentences of this one are clearly derived from
Galen's essay on the influence of the temperament or constitution of the body on the mind.[82]   Galen states that the
well-being of the mind will be furthered by the right use of
food, drink and other features of daily life, since the powers
or faculties of the mind depend on the temperament of the

body. We have been taught this, he adds, by Pythagoras, Plato and their followers.[83] (60b) Gaub refers to the Laws in his citation of Plato, but the same passage is quoted by Galen in the above-mentioned essay.[84]

XIII   The Variability of the Temperaments, and Its Source

62. Since the matter is self-evident it would be superfluous to add more instances. A consideration of the differences that mark off one healthy body from another is of more importance here. They are called the temperaments by physicians. Among men there is hardly less variation of temperaments than of faces, and their power over the mind is indeed very great. Between mind and body a certain degree of correspondence is to be seen, hence in accordance with differences of temperament the operations of the mind in various men are not of the same nature. Thus it has become a proverb that character accords with the temperament of the body.

63. Therefore, if the constitution of the body, the composition of the humors, the course of the circulation, and other corporeal activities are unique in a warm temperament, if all of these differ in a cold temperament and again in one moist or dry, no less great are the differences met with in particular features pertaining to the mind. You will look in vain for equality, either in power of understanding, force of judgement, acuteness of spirit, constancy of attention, tenacity of memory or fervor of imagination, in every temperament; you will seek in vain for the same inclinations, intensities, strengths and weaknesses. Just as in bodies so in minds, all of these differ.

64. There is surely no one who does not know this, since innumerable instances appear every day in the common life of man. Whether the primary source

should be looked for in the body or the mind, however, is indeed a disputed matter. The problem has greater scope and importance than I could possibly set forth here, let alone solve. Nevertheless I do not hesitate to say that when I compare the numerous and different parts composing the body with the great simplicity which it is proper to ascribe to the mind, it seems to me much more likely that the seat of this diversity—I will not say the sole, but the most important—lies in something which is by nature multiform. But not to stray further from my theme I shall be compliant and move along a path midway between different opinions, granting that just as much is due to the mind as to the body in this connection. Indeed, in my opinion those who hold that the body ought not be considered here at all take insufficient account of the frequency with which the faculties and habits of the mind are altered when age, illness, or any other such factor changes the bodily temperament.

65. I consider it plain, therefore, that the philosopher cannot dispense with the aid of the physician wheresoever the understanding of the human mind, or its improvement by precept, are concerned. Other than the physician, who will describe the particular temperament of any one person, who the mental capacities proper to any given temperament, who the emotions, desires and weaknesses of men's minds, which are of different force and kind in bodies differently constituted? Just as all fruits and trees are not to be found in every field, so all strengths and weaknesses do not arise in every temperament. Something good and something bad is present everywhere, but to a different degree in each case.

(62) Gaub now introduces the doctrine of the temperaments, a doctrine that has played a prominent part in medical thought from the time of its formulation by Galen in the second century A.D. down to the present day. The

temperaments are corporeal phenomena but at least since Galen they have been correlated with character, i.e. mental traits. The temperament exerts a powerful influence on the mind, and this fact, Gaub says, is the origin of the proverb that character accords with the temperament of the body.[85] The "proverb" is of course the Latin title of Galen's essay referred to above. (63) The composition of the solid and fluid components of the human body as well as the course of the natural and vital functions differ in the different temperaments. Gaub names the psychological strengths and weaknesses which are associated with and thought to be partly consequences of these corporeal differences. (64a) The correlation of mind with body, of character or behavior with bodily temperament, was generally recognized, as Gaub says, but there continued to be dispute regarding its "primary source". Does mind depend on body to a greater extent than body on mind or vice versa? The controversy has been a live one since the early days of Greek medicine, and the various conflicting views may be found in Plato.[86] As Gaub remarks, the problem is one of great scope and importance. He recognizes its bearing on the question of personal responsibility and will discuss this later. For his own part he believes in the simplicity or unity of the mind and, for reasons that are not clear, holds that the source of something complex and variable (in this case the character or behavior) must itself be complex and variable, as the body is. Note that he does not call it the only source, but simply the most important. (64b) Gaub's notion of the temperaments, in keeping with medical tradition, includes the belief that the temperament of any given individual is highly variable and subject to the changing influence of age, season, illness and use of the non-naturals. (65) Previously Gaub has told us (§4) that the early philosophers were physicians as well because they were aware of these inter-relationships.

XIV   Classification and Description
of the Temperaments

66. In that called the sanguine temperament an easily taught, ready, generous and flexible disposition is coupled with negligence, want of foresight, inconstancy, immoderacy and an unbridled love of pleasure.

67. In the melancholic constitution everything is the opposite. The understanding is slow but most penetrating, the power of attention is tireless and pursuit of whatever has been initiated is tenacious. They are prudent beyond measure, covetous and suspicious, and their emotions are sluggish indeed but hard to suppress.

68. You will praise the pungent spirit and glowing imagination, the fiery readiness for action and the steadfastness of the choleric man, but you will deplore the ready rashness to dare all, and the harsh irascibility and insufferable pride with which they are coupled.

69. Finally, shall I arouse the sleepy phlegmatics, unresponsive to everything, striving greatly for nothing, of whom it may be said that they live for their gullets and bellies alone?

70. Do you truly believe it of little importance, gentlemen, for the philosopher to learn this from the physician so that he may become thoroughly acquainted with his own temperament and the temperaments of those whom he takes under his tutelage—with what is good and bad, what is to be cultivated and cherished, what stifled and repressed?   This would be like saying that all plants require the same kind of care, or that all bodily ailments can be healed by one remedy.

71. But indeed I shall allow that these matters are of little importance and to an attentive observer are readily perceptible even without the physician's help. Nevertheless, if a remedy for the faults and affections

of the mind that are seated in the temperaments is to be had I believe it will be furnished by the physician or no one, as long as we do not abandon human powers.

72. I do not wish to detract completely from the usefulness and efficacy of reasoning, advising, admonishing and rebuking, of strict and earnest discipline, in this connection. They often help in preventing vices from forcibly breaking out. When the latter are fixed in the structure of the body, however, it is difficult to pluck them out in such a way that they do not return again and again. The root deeply seated in the body must be torn out. If it is left behind a new weed will spring up immediately even though you cut off the stalk.

73. Those to whom we entrust the task of directing men's minds to better ends very rarely consider remedies of this kind, and seldom apply them diligently and properly even when they are perhaps convinced of their usefulness. It can no longer seem too remarkable that they try so many unhappy remedies of their own, yet accomplish almost nothing when the constitution of the body is adverse. In the case of an Alcibiades not even the teachings of Socrates could prevail.

(66–69) Gaub mentioned four simple temperaments in §63: warm, cold, moist and dry, corresponding to the four primary qualities of the four elements. He now introduces the more familiar complex temperaments: choleric (warm and dry), melancholic (cold and dry), phlegmatic (cold and moist) and sanguine (moist and warm). We note that although Gaub regards the temperaments as corporeal phenomena he has little to say regarding their anatomical or physiological basis and limits himself to a description of the corresponding psychological traits. He wishes to direct the attention of his audience to this gap in medical theory (§77, 78). (71) The first sentence contains a rhetorical admission. In the second, human powers are contrasted by implication with divine powers. Gaub would probably admit that a man's temperament might be more readily modified by a divine act of grace than by moral exhortation. (72) Nevertheless, he does not wish to deny all efficacy to the use of words. In this paragraph there is an interesting inversion of Cicero's views expressed in the *Tusculan Disputations*. Cicero claims that the cure for diseases of the mind is to demonstrate to the afflicted person that his difficulties are the result of a mistaken belief, submission to which he considers to be right. This error (of the mind) is the root of all evil and philosophy promises to pull it out.[87] Gaub, on the other hand, claims that when vices are rooted in the structure of the body it is difficult to pluck them out in such a way that they do not recur again and again, since the root deeply seated in the *body* must be torn out.[88] (73) This allusion to Socrates also appears in a work attributed to Boerhaave, Gaub's teacher.[89]

XV   Imbalance and Variability of the Temperaments

74. Since there is some degree of intemperance in every temperament, capable of causing harm if it increases beyond bounds, certainly the concern of the physician is to check whatever is excessive by making proper use of the non-naturals and other aids, lest the health of the body be destroyed. In so doing why should he not be able to cure diseases of the mind having a like origin? What do I say? Is a cure to be hoped for other than from the physician?

75. When a drunken man rushes impetuously and blindly headlong into lechery or any other shameful act, would you rule him by reason and divert him from his madness while his body is still heated with wine? Or would you, rather, having removed the occasion of the offense, try to put the man to sleep as quickly as

possible, in order to rout the effects of wine that were the cause of the madness? Would you then attempt to shape his mind by precept so that even when drunk he will nonetheless shrink from vice? Or would you take care that in the future he does not drink wine in excess? Everyone can see, I think, that the happier effort will be directed at the body, since the mind is driven beside itself and aroused to a frenzy by a disturbance of the body. Is the account of the alterations induced in the understanding or will by the temperaments any different? I admit that the latter are extremely difficult to change. Yet it is even more difficult to give a new stamp to the mind when they are left unaltered. And it is wrong to withdraw diseases from the province of medicine because they are difficult to cure. Although it is not easy by any manner of means to mold or even to modify the constitution of the body so that it stays within modest bounds it is nevertheless not beyond all power of the medical art, provided that men will be sufficiently earnest and persistent in the application of whatever may be of use.

76. That men shift from one temperament to another through the influence of age or disease, or even because of a change in mode of life, is an everyday observation. Hence nothing prevents the physician from being able also to bring about similar changes through his own procedures. It is well known that the excesses to which all temperaments whatsoever are prone are made worse by wrong modes of life and not uncommonly amount to disease. Indeed most of them are given greater intensity by an overabundance of blood alone. Who would wish to deny that there are means to blunt even if not to divert their overwhelming force and weaken their onslaught? Since it is excess in these things that chiefly harms the mind, disturbing and dulling the intelligence and bending the will toward vice but making it hesitant before virtue, I consider it

quite plain that to seek aid from the physician against these mental hindrances is neither idle nor useless but rather a matter of prime necessity. If you hold that authorities have a place here, gentlemen, one Galen, equally outstanding as physician and philosopher, is worth all the rest. In dealing with the subject he does not hesitate to say with great confidence: "Now, therefore, those who were unwilling to admit that nutriments may make men more or less temperate, licentious, unruly, discrete, bold, timid, gentle, and lovers or partakers of quarrels and brawls, should be reasonable enough to come to me to learn what to eat and drink! For in this way they will be greatly helped toward moral philosophy. They will, moreover, make progress toward the attainment of moral strength and become more perceptive, retentive, prudent and eager to learn, to the advantage of the rational faculties of the mind. In addition to the foods and drinks I shall also teach them the winds, climates and regions whose use is to be avoided or sought out."

77. Would that this aspect of medicine, from which so much of value to mankind and of honor and renown to physicians might be hoped for, were not so undeveloped that it can only be called neglected! If you look at what is commonly held today concerning variations of temperaments, it consists only of not very helpful generalities and minutiae, as incapable of embracing their infinite variety as a nutshell the *Iliad*. Although there has been long and ceaseless discussion of the various states of the body and its parts that characterize, determine, and pertain to any one of the temperaments, nevertheless what we have is too uncertain and poorly defined to be of much use in practice. Lastly, although the proper handling of the temperaments ought to have been a primary concern of physicians, to our regret we labor here under an even greater lack with regard to pertinent matters.

But it will suffice to touch lightly on this, not to incommode you. Men versed in these things know how much is wanting in the medical doctrine of the temperaments that would, if it were thoroughly investigated and explained through painstaking observation, certainly aid the physician in the whole scope of his art, particularly so in the part of which I speak.

78. Is it not a worn commonplace that men undergo not only great physical but also great mental changes as they move gradually through the various stages of life? How greatly different is the youth from the old man and the child from the adult in faculties of understanding, in thought, judgement and memory, in bent of the will, in behavior and impulse! How far the sexes are apart in this respect! Compare different nations and peoples among themselves! Here too you will find an unbelievable diversity of faculties and affections of the mind. Englishmen, Spaniards, Italians, French and other peoples are stamped by their peculiar features, nor do the same strengths or weaknesses prevail among all. "The Scythians have only one philosopher, but in Athens there are many; numerous Abderites, again, are feeble-minded, but few Athenians." It seemed to Plato that the source of the discrepancy ought to be attributed in part to differences in sun and climate. "The Goddess", he adds, "in founding Athens chose a region that would give birth to the most sagacious spirits, in consequence of its tempered climate. The wise and warlike Goddess considered that a region should be chosen such as to bring forth men like herself." How one man differs from another when he has been more gently or harshly treated, and has become accustomed to a different way of life, especially from boyhood on! How greatly is a man's mind, even when it remains sound, sometimes altered by bodily disease! One may almost doubt that it is the same. Not without

reason do the folk consider this a bad sign and its opposite, when the sick man returns to himself, a good one. Before regaining their strength men recovering from illness sometimes find their affections, habits and desires very different from those to which they were accustomed when fully healthy; they are, as it were, strangers to and ignorant of themselves! I have known those to whom irascibility from this cause was so disagreeable—although disgusted with themselves they were nevertheless unable with the aid of reason alone to keep their rage from repeatedly boiling over— that when their mental balance was finally restored, together with their strength, they congratulated themselves more on this than on recovery from bodily disease.

79. To what end all of this? Only so that you will understand, gentlemen, that the manifold dissimilarity of minds is in large part due to diversities of the temperaments, and hence that physicians will understand more accurately, explain more clearly and cure more happily only when they at last achieve a fuller view of the nature of the temperaments.

(74a) Every temperament has its peculiar type of excess or imbalance,[90] inclining it in a particular direction. The physician must operate within a system of checks and balances for the benefit of the patient, appropriately regulating his food and drink, sleeping and waking, retention and evacuation, movement and rest, and states of mind (the six non-naturals). Only in this way can health be maintained and, says Gaub, diseases of the mind[91] having "a like origin" cured. In order to understand the significance of Gaub's remarks regarding "intemperance" we must bear in mind that the bodily temperaments in Galenical medicine are states of *imbalance* rather than balance. The early Greek view, or at least a prevailing one, seems to have been that health represented a dynamic state of balance of the elements, humors and qualities,[92] but in Galen correct balance is regarded as of very unusual occurrence. Galen describes four simple and four compound states of imbalance, i.e. eight temperaments, and argues that these presuppose a ninth and perfectly balanced temperament.[93] The associated character traits are briefly indicated in another Galenical treatise.[94] (74b) The kind of intemperance for which Gaub uses the Latin term *intemperies* is a corporeal phenomenon, i.e. a state of corporeal imbalance. It should be distinguished from intemperance of the mind (which, however, may be partly dependent on it). Cicero writes that what the Greeks call *sôphrosynê* he calls temperance or moderation.[95] This "sôphrosynê" is temperance of mind, not of body. Cicero compares the two types of temperance (for which we have two names in Greek, but only one in Latin) as follows: the congruence of the various virtues of the body is called the temperance of health, just as the concord of beliefs and judgements is called temperance of the mind.[96] (75) We have here a reduction to the absurd of the "philosopher's" position. The drunken man behaves badly only when drunk. Should we attempt so to shape his mind by precept that he will behave well even when he is drunk? Gaub has told us that the physician is properly concerned with the mind in two sets of circumstances: (1) when the mental derangement is due to a deranged state of the body or can be alleviated by action taken on the body, (2) when the mind is the cause of the bodily disease or when bodily disease can be alleviated by action taken on the mind. He argues here that the more practicable mode of treatment is that taken against the body. The patient should be kept sober (he overlooks the difficulties). This apparently banal example introduces a problem of fundamental importance. Everyone admits that here a disturbance of the body, induced by wine, has driven the mind into a frenzy. But, asks Gaub, are not all affections of the mind likewise due to variations in the constitution of the body, and is it not futile to attempt to control them without taking this into account? It is not beyond the power of the medical art to alter the make-up of the body, he adds, although it is admittedly a difficult task. (76a) Gaub emphasizes again that the temperament of a man, the constitution of the solid and fluid components of his body, fluctuates and is subject to the influences of age, season, disease and mode of life. This had been more or less standard medical doctrine for a very long time and had remained so in spite of the changes introduced into the theory of the temperaments by Gaub's day. Some early ideas on these influences may be found in the treatise on the humors attributed to Galen.[97] (76b) Gaub's remark that all temperaments are prone to excesses which may become severe enough, in consequence of a wrong mode of life, to amount to disease is perhaps not entirely consistent with his statement elsewhere that disturbances of the bodily functions due to age, sex and temperament should not be classified as diseases.[98] (76c) Gaub cites Galen's essay on the influence of bodily temperament on mental faculties at this point (see Note 5). The quotation should be compared with that from Descartes contained in §50. Descartes's proposal is less specific but more far-reaching, since he does not limit himself to the potential effects of diet and climate. (76d) The ultimate sources of Galen's ideas on the subject of the far-reaching effects of diet are probably both Pythagorean and Empedoclean. The Pythagoreans believed that every kind of food or drink, of which wine was only the most obvious example, was responsible for a certain characteristic turn of the mind.[99] If this had implied that mental traits were fully determined by physical factors, it would have meant the end of personal responsibility when carried to the extreme. One of Galen's more proximate and most important sources was the *Timaeus* of Plato. Timaeus states at one point that the wicked are wrongly reproached, for no one is voluntarily wicked but rather becomes so because of an evil condition of the body (due to) poor nurture. His explanation of how this occurs is that the humors of the body become deranged and mingle their vapour with the movement of the *psyche*, thus implanting in it diseases of all kinds, varying in intensity and extent. Hence we may say that the wicked become so from involuntary

causes.[100]   Taylor claims that the whole of this section
of the *Timaeus* is an attempt to graft Empedoclean
materialistic psychology on Pythagorean doctrines, an error
in principle the fruit of which was the doctrine that the
psychê is no more than a reflection of the harmony or crasis
of the bodily constituents.[101]   (77a) Gaub no longer
believes in the four-element theory that was the basis of the
original doctrine of the temperaments, nor in the details of
Galenical physiology.   The advances in anatomy, physiology and chemistry had carried medicine beyond this
point.   The "infinite variety" of the temperaments, however, had not been embraced by the newer knowledge.
(77b) Gaub does not seem to grasp clearly the double
meaning of temperament, corporeal *krasis* on the one hand
and mental *sôphrosynê* on the other, although the distinction
would have been very much in keeping with his dualism.
(78a) Gaub's remarks should be understood in a general
sense, without reference to older theories, but it is interesting
to note the comments of the writer of the Galenical medical
definitions on this topic.   He likens the four ages of man,
adolescence, youth, middle age, and old age, to the four
seasons.   Spring and adolescence (the period of growth)
are hot and moist, youth and summer are hot and dry,
autumn and middle age are cold and dry, winter and old
age, cold and moist.[102]   (78b) Gaub now quotes first from
Galen's *Quod animi mores corporis temperamenta sequantur*
(see Note 5) and then from the *Timaeus*.   (79) Mental
diversity has its roots in corporeal diversity, in other words
sôphrosynê is rooted in *krasis*.   Until physicians understand
the physical basis of man's behavior they will be unable to
manage or control it.[103]

XVI True Diseases of the Mind Differentiated from Relatively Minor Disturbances

80. I come now to those defects of the mind customarily and rightly reckoned among diseases. If a man is afflicted by one of them we say that he is ill. Although the affections of the mind discussed above properly ought to be considered illnesses there is no mortal so happy that he does not suffer from some one of them, and a gentler name is therefore widely accepted lest all of us be considered of unsound mind. And, indeed, where everyone is a Polyphemus, who will censure the one-eyed man?

81. Many of these diseases of the mind, it is true, so plainly arise from a weakened state of the body that all acknowledge their treatment to fall within the province of the physician. I refer to mania, melancholy, phrenitis, febrile delirium, nymphomania, rabies from the bites of rabid animals, catalepsy, and so forth. Since there is neither doubt nor dispute here I shall say no more, in order not to seem deliberately and rashly long-winded.

82. I very often marvel that there is no one who does not freely admit that all diseases of this kind belong in the medical forum when they are preceded or accompanied by some obvious bodily defect known by everyone to have produced a disturbance in the mind—whether because the disturbance immediately followed the defect, or because the body was at the same time even more violently and seriously affected than the mind, or because the ailment rapidly involved all faculties of the mind, or yet because we have been taught by repeated observation that such affections of the body often derange the mind. Yet where circumstances of this kind are lacking the aid of the physician is rarely sought, even though the diseases

are the same, and when it is at last, only after many useless and wrongly applied, not to say harmful, measures have permitted them to strike roots so deep that they cannot be wholly removed. As if here, too, there could not be bodily causes of unusual or less obvious nature, such as to bring about a change in the body recognizable by nothing other than mental illness, or that slowly, secretly, and step by step steals in on the body by degrees.

(80) The terminology becomes very involved at this point, Gaub speaks first of those "defects of the mind" properly and ordinarily considered "diseases"; if a man is afflicted by one of them "we say that he is ill".[104] The "affections of the mind" previously discussed (anger, and strong emotions in general) are themselves a kind of "sickness", he claims, but since all of us at one time or another become sick in this sense a milder term is used, lest we all be "considered of unsound mind".[105] The point is that Gaub prefers not to stigmatize the emotional disturbances which are the common lot of man with the terms "disease", "sickness" or "illness", the more so since these terms can serve to designate the severe and lasting disturbances of the mind briefly indicated in the next paragraph. (81) The diseases of the mind referred to here are the severe defects mentioned above and presumably include what would today be called the major and minor psychoses, some of the more severe neuroses, and a number of organic diseases involving the brain. Some of these, Gaub says, plainly arise from a weakened state of the body.[106] Mania and melancholy (the disease melancholy, not the transient state of mind) were looked on as the consequence of prolonged severe imbalance of the humors. Phrenitis was the designation of an acute fever associated with inflammation of the meninges of the brain, leading to mental disturbances.[107] Nymphomania or "uterine furors", as Gaub calls it, was thought to have an organic or corporeal basis. (See Note 126, second lecture, for a seventeenth-century discussion.)

99

Catalepsy is defined by a standard eighteenth-century medical dictionary as "loss of vision with open eyes".[108]   (82) Gaub has no more to say of these diseases, since everyone is convinced already that they have a corporeal basis.   When bodily disease is thought to be at the root of a mental disturbance—as in the case of phrenitis for example—everyone admits that the patient belongs in the hand of a physician. But why, Gaub asks, should we suppose that the bodily disease or underlying corporeal defect must be immediately obvious?   May some abnormalities generally considered to involve the mind only have subtle corporeal causes? Gaub suggests that the corporeal changes may be so hidden as to manifest themselves only in the form of mental derangement.

XVII   Illustrative Cases of Mental Disturbances Due to Corporeal Defects

83. Olaus Borrichius tells of a dull and blunt-spirited youth who was able to learn almost nothing, although he had the services of the same teacher as did a brother who was well advanced in his studies. Seized by a malignant fever he began, after much raving, on the third day of the disease to hold forth like someone quite sound on the vanity of the world, on contempt of death, and on scorn for the dissolution of the body, with as much erudition as unexpected eloquence—all of this without a trace of madness and in a way that no learned son of Seneca could have bettered.   Shortly thereafter he again became delirious and expired.   Perhaps some will believe that this mental change ought to be attributed to a higher cause. I have no desire to oppose them if they will grant in turn that the mental change was the result of a bodily change and that the fever was no less the occasion of wisdom than of folly.

84. Many years ago I saw a woman who had for a

long time been greatly saddened by the dissolute life of her husband. On the advice of certain old wives she at last sought in brandy drinking both for solace and, in particular, for courage to give her man a thorough scolding. Indeed she found both, but this as well, that whenever she served Bacchus she lost, in the most pitiable fashion, all hope of the eternal salvation of her soul. I recall the numerous arguments, the repeated exhortations, and the many attempts at consolation tried in vain before the cause and cure of the recurring affliction was discovered in a woman who, considering her otherwise upright behavior, would scarcely have been suspected of inebriety.

85. In a certain nearby city careful observation disclosed that a matron was overcome by an ungovernable compulsion to steal when pregnant. She lacked nothing whatsoever, yet she was unable to keep herself from secretly making away with whatever property of others that came her way, even the silverware of her friends at whose banquets she was received. After delivery she was free of the compulsion, but with each successive pregnancy she was overcome anew, and moreover she even transmitted the unhappy inheritance to some of her children.

86. Shall I recall the women driven by abnormal appetites during pregnancy to such a point of inhumanity that they did not shrink from killing not only strangers but even their own husbands and eating their flesh? Although this condition is quite rare and extraordinary everyone will, I believe, agree that since it occurs during pregnancy—and remarkable instances of perversions of the appetite arising from this source present themselves on all sides—it ought to be attributed to the gravid uterus and hence to the body. Nevertheless, the opinion of the judges with respect to the similar case of Elizabeth of Milan was different and much harsher. Being subject to a disease of this kind, it seems, she would entice children away with

promises, lead them to her home for slaughter, preserve their flesh in brine and eat of it daily. We read that she perished under the torture of the wheel and fire. But should guilt have been ascribed to the mind rather than the body because the uterus of this woman happened not to have been gravid? As if other causes arising from weakness could not excite perverted appetites also, as if infants, virgins, old women and even men did not sometimes suffer from them! A Scottish girl who was the daughter of a cannibalistic robber was no better used by fate. Hardly more then twelve years old she was caught in her father's crime and, in accordance with an extremely harsh sentence, condemned to be buried alive. Yet she had lost her parents, both of whom were burned, when she was hardly a year old. From that time on she had been raised by others, and it therefore seems most likely that the monstrous appetite of the parents was inborn and transmitted to the unhappy offspring by an hereditary taint.

87. I gladly pass over many other virtues and vices rooted, as it were, in the seed and through its influence not uncommonly transmitted from ancestors to a long succession of descendants, becoming to some extent characteristic of a family. I also omit those implanted in the fetus through commerce with the mother. Nor shall I recall how often the mind of a wellborn infant is corrupted by the milk of an immoral wet-nurse and inclined toward vices of the worst kind, completely foreign to its family stock. Anyone who wishes to search the observations of physicians will uncover many pertinent cases, and almost no one is so inexperienced that his memory will not furnish an example, since even in friendly conversations it happens that the discussion turns by chance toward this topic.

88. Indeed, since one and all of the instances mentioned here are so in agreement, to deny that spread from the body to the mind had taken place

would be absurd, although to explain just how this comes about would be very difficult. Hence it is no longer possible for anyone to doubt that, in general, there are agencies apparently having the power of acting on the body alone but capable of bringing about tremendous changes in the mind as well, although this power may not be very great and may at times hardly suffice to damage the body at all or to affect it in any obviously perceptible way. Why should this seem surprising to anyone when the parts of the body that serve the workings of the mind are of a fineness that mocks the extent of man's industry and intelligence? Hence the most careful scrutiny of the bodies of men whose actions while they lived were extremely disturbed usually discloses nothing whatsoever that is corrupted or departs significantly from normal.

89. Further, no one is unaware, I believe, that something purely corporeal and borne by thousands of men with impunity may nevertheless cause at times in a certain individual—in whom you cannot observe that his body is so peculiarly fashioned—the most serious alterations of the faculties of the mind, alterations that surpass the human understanding.

(83) Olaus Borrichius (Ole Borch) was a seventeenth-century Danish polymath.[109] The story of the dull-witted youth does not advance Gaub's argument, since the boy's startling mental transformation was associated with an obvious corporeal disturbance, but it does show that the latter is not necessarily accompanied by a mental defect. The topic of the "learned discourse" was a favorite of the Stoics. (84) Argument, exhortation and consolation, the mainstays of "philosophical" treatment were bound to fail, according to Gaub, as long as the corporeal determining factor, i.e. the effects of wine on the woman's body, remained hidden. We see that what appears to be a problem in homiletics reveals itself as a problem in toxicology or pathological metabolism. A theologian might reasonably

object that inebriety had simply uncovered the woman's religious problem, and that the apparent cure on withdrawing alcohol was in reality no more than the masking of a theological "disease". Gaub would retort that ultimate causes are no concern of the physician, and that if the complaint disappears when what the physician takes to be the cause is withdrawn he asks no more. (85) The unwilling mind is drawn into wickedness by the brute body, as Gaub remarked in §6. The causal connection between bodily state and moral behavior in this case of pregnancy kleptomania meets his requirements.[110] (86) Gaub cites Schenck von Grafenberg, a sixteenth-century physician of Freiburg, as the source of his second case.[111] According to this account the woman voluntarily confessed her crime and asked to be punished. She was sentenced to life imprisonment. The mildness of her sentence suggests that her judges did not regard her as fully responsible. Gaub cites Bugati's *Universal History* as the source of the case of Elizabeth of Milan. It can also be found in Donatus, where it is attributed to Bugati and described in much the same words as those used by Gaub in recounting the story.[112] Donatus, a physician, believed, as did Gaub, that Elizabeth was suffering from a compulsive unnatural appetite (pica) that limited her moral responsibility.[113] Donatus also reports the case of the Scottish girl and comments that she went to her living grave still unrepentant, proclaiming that no one would abstain from human flesh if he once learned how delicious it was.[114] In speaking of Elizabeth, Gaub uses the phrase "subject to a disease of this kind" because he wishes to emphasize that a corporeal disease rather than moral failure was at the root of her abnormal behavior.[115] In the case of the Scottish girl he finds that the evidence suggests a corporeal taint "rooted in the seed", to anticipate his words in the next paragraph. He has already mentioned a possible instance of this kind in §85. (87) The belief that an infant might not only be physically but morally poisoned by the milk of a wet-nurse (or mother) was fairly widely held in Gaub's time. For a discussion of the way in which this may come about see the commentary to Gaub II, 18. (88) Gaub points to the central role of the nervous system in connection with the problem of how agencies primarily affecting the body may produce even greater secondary changes in the mind. It is not clear whether the phrase, "fineness that mocks the power of man's industry and intelligence" refers to the fine structure of the brain (of which relatively little was known in his day) or to the complexity of the peripheral nervous system—the "neural man" of §39. The fineness of the anatomical changes occurring in the mentally ill account, he claims, for the fact that so little is found at autopsy. (89) The nature of the purely corporeal agencies referred to here is not mentioned. We observe, Gaub writes in his textbook, that men are unequally affected by similar agents. In explaining the reason for this he distinguishes predisposing from occasional causes of disease. The former are inherent, persisting, states of the body. Disease may occur when occasional causes (broadly speaking, the abuse of the non-naturals[116]) cooperate, but if the predisposing causes are absent the corresponding occasional causes are ineffective.[117] Diseases of allergy and food idiosyncrasies immediately come to mind, but Gaub evidently refers here to something having to do with mental derangement.

XVIII   Delay in Treating the Bodily Cause of a Mental Ailment is Dangerous

90. Whenever the mind is so indisposed that a bodily cause of censure seems absent one should, therefore, not at once conclude that the disease is beyond the power of the medical art and that since it is brought about by non-bodily causes it requires remedies of like nature. To determine with certainty whether the mind is suffering on its own account or that of the body is actually much more difficult than many people suppose. Whoever closely considers the instances and

proofs that I have presented above will surely be forced to admit, unless everything deceives me, that even when there is no obvious bodily affection something hidden may nevertheless quite frequently be present. As long as we are uncertain of, and in fact cannot ascertain, the side of man on which the disease originates is it not plain to everyone that it will be more prudent to take measures toward altering the body? If the latter is overlooked and all treatment is directed solely toward the mind we run the danger that if by chance the disease is corporeal it will in the end, after having prevailed for a time, become chronic and utterly resist appropriate treatment, although it might easily have been dealt with in the beginning. Nor can it be objected that a similar danger will arise when, on the other hand, the mind perhaps turns out to be the weak point. This is so far from being the case that emotional disturbances not continually furnished tinder and breathed on by the body neither grow worse with delay nor are forcefully urged by their own impetus to take root more deeply. Rather do we see them of their own accord grow weaker and weaker and finally disappear.

91. Lastly, if at times there do occur ailments of the mind so pure and so remote from the body that it clearly seems no role should be ascribed to the latter, I venture nevertheless to say that even in such instances medical counsel will be of value. For just as disturbances of the body are readily transmitted to the mind so, on the other hand, when the latter is disordered the health of the bodily parts does not long remain unimpaired. What were at first simple ailments of the mind alone, without any cause or contribution from elsewhere, gradually pass over into the body and by deranging its activities win and heap up substance, as it were, for nourishment so that they may not only be supported and fostered for a long time but may even be provoked to become worse. So frequently does

this occur among hypochondriacs and melancholics that it has given rise among physicians to those well-known phrases, according to which some are said to suffer "with matter" and others "without matter".

92. I consider it plain, therefore, and for more than one reason, that at least some of these ailments also pertain to the field of medicine. For even when the injury is still fresh the body ought to be protected lest it be drawn into the illness by effective intercourse with the afflicted mind and then repeatedly aggravate the latter with fresh attacks. Once established it is clear that all remedies whatsoever will be applied in vain unless the already accumulated and continually increasing material basis is expelled. A cure of the mind cannot be expected in the face of repeated onslaughts from a persisting ailment of the body.

(90) Here is a clear statement of what has been implied previously on several occasions, that it is the duty of the physician to rule out all possible corporeal causes of mental ailments, and that to do this is much more difficult than many people suppose. In any doubtful case the physician should first direct his attention to the body, since delay may allow the corporeal cause, if present, to strike root too deeply for later removal. Gaub claims that delay is less dangerous when the cause of the mental disturbance lies in the mind itself, for such disturbances often disappear of their own accord unless they develop a corporeal basis. (91a) Even "pure diseases of the mind" may require the physician's care, firstly because measures taken against the body may be the most effective, and secondly, because the interaction of mind and body may allow the ailment to establish a foothold in the body. This would seem to contradict the rationale of the therapeutic directive given in the previous paragraph, since the establishment of a foothold would obviously be favored by delay. (91b) Gaub mentions the "well-known" phrases "with matter" and "without matter".[118] In the same way a modern physician might

speak of neurotic disorders with or without an organic component. Gaub's "well-known phrases" are attributed to Galen in Kühn's study of his medical system, although in a slightly different sense. Galen distinguished diseases of the organs and of similar parts. The latter were due to imbalance of the humors (*dyscrasia*) of which there were two varieties, one "with matter" and one "without it".[119] Too much or too little of one of the qualities gave rise to those "without matter" (a dynamic disturbance, as it were), while in those "with matter" there was an abnormal accumulation of humors in the part affected.[120] Gaub may be interpreted here to mean that a long-standing mental or emotional disturbance may produce a local lesion due to a derangement of the humors, although his "humors" are not to be equated with those of Galen. (92) The ailments referred to here are those which at first sight appear to have no corporeal cause. Gaub restates his reasons for bringing them to the attention of the physician, which are: (1) the physician should protect the body against the onslaught of an afflicted mind, (2) he should prevent the establishment of a material basis for the mental disturbance.

XIX   The Physician Can Offer Symptomatic Relief for Mental Ailments by Treating the Body

93. Moreover, even the two parts that I have just mentioned do not entirely exhaust the role of the physician and all of the aid for which he is properly responsible in these diseases. As I have already pointed out above, we are taught by experience that the mind has differing perceptions in accordance with variations in the state of the body to which she is joined, hence the latter may interfere with her activities. At one time she is unable to think as she desires and at another she is forced, so to speak, to think what the body commands. Making proper use of this mutual linkage, the

physician can indeed apply his remedies in such a way as to give relief to a mental ailment even in the absence of any idea as to its causes or effects, present or feared, in the body.

94. At hand among the instruments of his art are those which will quiet the violently agitated mind, which will tear loose a mind fast bound to some particular subject, which will force her to rest by effacing thought and temporarily inducing oblivion. Do you doubt this? Then you do not know that all of these things can be accomplished by giving a narcotic and thereby lulling the body into a profound slumber.

95. Physicians have in their hands means to recall the mind when she has withdrawn herself from the body, to arouse and return her to herself when thought has ceased, or at least when awareness of thought has been lost, to stir her up when turned within and too intent upon herself, and to expel overfixed ideas and substitute others in their place. Such is the power of the stimulants that stir up the humors, excite the nerves, and inflict pain. How numerous and various are those that abound in the art of medicine!

96. Of them all I shall call attention here to but one, and that the most powerful. The most deeply seated mental defects and the most incurable forms of madness may sometimes be rooted out by anxiety—whether because the tormented and frightened mind is revived by the terrible punishment of her greatly depressed senses, or because she is thoroughly stirred up, inwardly moved and shaken to her depths everywhere by the struggle and imbued with a new spirit, or for some other reason. It is known that men with minds held captive by the violence of love or grief have, after accidentally falling into water and being thought dead for a time, been restored to life by careful treatment and have at the same time recovered full soundness of mind. It appears, however, that water is not the cause of the unexpected recovery, but rather the

frightful torment that the near loss of life from suffocation inflicts on the mind. This observation stimulated physicians not to leave untouched a path to the cure of diseases of the mind that chance had revealed. Thus was submersion therapy discovered and introduced into medicine, a terrible remedy indeed but one hardly to be exceeded in efficacy by any other when an unsound mind is to be helped by the effects of a bodily change. That many good results have been obtained in England has also been attested to by Helmont.

(93) In the absence of any sure knowledge of corporeal causes or effects it remains within the power of the physician to afford symptomatic relief in mental disorders, using drugs which act primarily on the body and secondarily on the mind. This paragraph seems phrased so as to call attention to the theoretical significance, with respect to his thesis that the mind can be influenced via the body, of the effect of narcotics. (94) The reference here is not necessarily to drugs, as we learn from the following paragraph. (95) A reference is now made to the use of pain in the treatment of mental ailments, but the point is not elaborated. (96) In this discussion of "submersion therapy" Gaub cites Franciscus van Helmont.[121] He attributes the cure to anxiety (see discussion of this topic in the commentary to §30).

XX Physicians Should Actively Engage in a Search for New Drugs Capable of Affecting the Mind

97. It seems to me, gentlemen, that I have now set forth the chief features of that regimen which I selected as the subject of my discourse. I could add much more that follows from what has been said. But your patience, which I know and regret that I have too much abused, forbids me to touch on these matters.

Prudence demands rather that I leave their discovery to your own ingenuity.

98. Yet before I end my discourse, be moved by my words, o all you physicians who labor with me in the healing art! That care of the human mind with which I have dealt is our concern; it is the noblest part of our calling, and the more diligently each of us cultivates it the more he will be worthy of the name of physician-philosopher and likewise of being deemed *isotheos*, in the words of Hippocrates. For if unconditional and complete health of the body is that which communicates itself to the mind, putting no hindrances in her way so that she is no less completely ready for wisdom than virtue, we ought to state plainly that the most desirable treatment for the body is one that at the same time helps the mind. Nor will our art be finished and perfected until it can make men not only as robust but also as superior in character and behavior as possible. Since we are forced to the painful admission that this aspect of the healing art has for a long time suffered from the most serious deficiencies and even now lies so neglected, ignored and alone that almost everything is wanting—although everywhere else great ardor is currently now being expended—take action, o my friends, and with experiments, observations, trials and whatever else may be of help in the effort collected in common, cultivate, embellish and perfect this medical philosophy! The worth of the topic demands, the progress of our art suggests, and the love of humanity requires that we attack this task and keep at it until we discover special regimens, universal therapeutic methods, and particular remedies with which we can awaken, sharpen or strengthen any faculty of the mind whatsoever, and moderate, arouse or repress its paroxysms, instincts and propensities as needed. Does the magnitude of the task strike terror? In other situations this is so far from depressing the mind as to enkindle it rather. Nor, indeed, should anyone

who carefully considers the few facts known from observation venture to call the task insuperable. Consider only how much fever is capable of altering the mind, I say! Since the chief effect lies in a change in the circulation of the humors, is it not very likely that diets and remedies to some degree arousing, checking or otherwise influencing the circulation could be no less effective? Further, how much an increase or decrease in the amount of blood! It is well known that the memory is weakened by blood loss, nor does it regain its integrity until the damage is made good. That anger, ferocity and lust are stirred up by an excess of blood and calmed by its withdrawal is now well established. No less wholesome than unusual, therefore, was the procedure of that physician, mentioned by Naudé, who is said to have so weakened his hot and lustful wife through repeated venesections and similar procedures carried out under the pretext of fear, that he was then easily able to win the cold and weakened woman away from illicit intercourse. For if it is quite plain that universal remedies of this kind have great power over the activities of the mind, experience teaches us that specific drugs have even more. I shall not recall that venerable remedy, too little understood today, the *nêpenthe* of Helen. Yet consider the astonishing and far too well known effects of wine! Indeed, they are so far-reaching that whoever knows how to use them properly seems able to dominate men's minds at will. I omit mention of opium, at whose twofold power with respect to wine we marvel even the more since it is effective in such small amounts. I say nothing of a somewhat similar seed from a plant of Malabar called *ganscho*, the fumes of which are supposed to induce a delightful intoxication when breathed in through the mouth and nose, inspiring soldiers with mettle and priests with ecstasy. Nor shall I describe that offensive ointment with which the wise women, as they are called, rub their bodies to fall into a profound stupor invariably accompanied by the same vision of having been transported after a long aerial journey into a distant place where they intermingle, cohabit and dance with others of their ilk, all of this being so firmly impressed on their fancy that no argument after they awake can convince them that it was an empty dream.   I pass over many other matters that would require another hour's time were I to treat of them here.   What little I have presented shows well enough, I believe, that it would be a happy and fruitful endeavor for some far-sighted persons to occupy themselves with a subject of such importance.

(97) The "regimen" referred to is, of course, that of the correct management of the mind by way of the body, i.e. the medical management of moral problems.   (98a) Gaub closes his talk with what might well pass as a manifesto for psychopharmacology.   He calls for a concerted effort by physicians to discover agents acting primarily on the body yet capable of arousing, repressing or otherwise modifying all faculties of the mind whatsoever.   The physician will then be worthy of the name of philosopher as well, indeed he will be godlike (*isotheos*).   (98b) The phrase "the physician-philosopher is equal to the gods" occurs in the Hippocratic essay *On Decorum*.[122]   The philosophy or wisdom referred to in the context of that essay is of entirely ethical character, it has nothing to do with natural philosophy.   Its ideal is *sôphrosynê*: modesty, reserve, sound judgement and knowledge of the good.   The writer does not say that these virtues are to be obtained via the medical management of the body.   Gaub, on the other hand, asks for medical means to better men's minds and characters (recall the quotations from Descartes in §50 and Galen in §76), the medical means comprising drugs and all other corporeally acting agents, including those falling in the category of the non-naturals.   (98c) His illustrations are considerably less novel.   The statement that memory is weakened by blood loss is supported by a reference to the contemporary

literature.[123]   In spite of the remark regarding the unusual treatment carried out by Naudé's physician,[124] bleeding is mentioned by Perdulcis as a routine procedure in nymphomania.[125]   The *nêpenthe* of Helen has been the subject of much controversy.   In his essay on behavior and the bodily temperament Galen refers to the drug in passing as "the root of *oinopia*".   In a note to the translation of this essay Daremberg states that *nêpenthe* has been supposed to be opium, datura or hashish.   As for "oinopia" nothing is known of such a plant.[126]   "Ganscho" is no doubt a corruption of *ganja* (Indian hemp or *Cannabis activa*).   The flying ointments used by witches are said to have contained aconite, belladonna and hemlock in varying mixture, all being powerful drugs capable of producing mental confusion or delirium.[127]

Essay of 1763

I   Julien La Mettrie's *Man a Machine*

1. I believe, gentlemen, that you will be astonished when I announce that in this anniversary day of our University, the celebration of which requires from me a public oration, I intend to discuss again the same topic that I dealt with on this platform sixteen years ago, when retiring from the rectorate for the first time. What!—do I dare to serve up a warmed-over repast? I shall make you the intrepid judges of whether or not I am capable of sinking to this level.   Does the wealth of material therefore—not exhausted even by a discussion prolonged to the point of tedium—demand a sequel?   I hope that you, no less than I, feel that enough has been said for those of discernment!   Or am I rather minded to sing a recantation, to withdraw on second thought that which was perhaps vague or insufficiently considered and once escaped inadvertently?   I do indeed regret bitterly that a little Frenchman—a Mimus or Momus?—brought forth a repulsive offspring, to wit, his mechanical man, not long after sitting before this chair and hearing me speak, and did this in such a way that it seemed to many people that I had furnished him with, if not sparks for his flame, at least matter for embellishing his monstrosity.   I dismiss inquiry whether this should be considered more true than false.   I admit its relative truth.   Who will make the fault mine, however, that the impudence of a wanton spirit has defiled what I innocently offered to the public, not with reasoning but with the most senseless kind of raillery?   As if it were proper to condemn a food as unwholesome because it was corrupted into bile by a disturbed

115

stomach! Indeed it has been known for a long time that nothing can be asserted so true, so in accord with right reason, and, finally, so sacred, that the worst sort of petty philosophers will not venture to abuse it in order to decorate the fabrications of their fancy. Lest I seem to attract rather than repel blame with superfluous excuses let me add only that, in accordance with medical custom, I spoke carefully and in good faith to my fellow physicians about a topic of medical dispute, on the basis of detailed observations both of my own and others. I searched out and set forth views of nature; since they were established with that degree of certainty in understanding the works of nature beyond which the human intelligence cannot go, I am in no way led to discover any reason why I should retract an opinion or fear the stern rod of the censor.

2. Lest you be kept overlong in suspense by my introductory remarks, I shall now banish your doubts and disclose the topic of which I propose to treat today. Although it may seem identical with the former it is in truth not only different but also such that it cannot be regarded as unworthy of this assemblage which I am bound to respect, of your silence, whose favor I ask, or, finally, of the personage whom this day sets over me. I shall speak, certainly, on the management of the mind as it concerns physicians, but since I have already shown that it falls into two parts, only the first of which I have discussed, I am resolved so to speak as to follow up as far as possible the second, which it was necessary to pass over at that time. You will see, gentlemen, that I shall now set forth the wards of health coming to the body from the mind, since I have already dealt with the care of the body through which the mind flourishes.

3. If, as is customary, I undertook to draw your favor by commending the excellence of the subject, I fear that I should seem instead to hold less than a fitting opinion of your judgements, and that the more I

extolled it the more you would be led to suspect the slightness of the speaker. Relying solely on your courtesy, therefore, which has attended me whenever I have had occasion to speak in this place, I pray and beseech you to grant me your tongues and ears for this hour. For when I obtain this from you, even though a meagre style of speaking may perhaps detract from the merits of the subject, you will nevertheless reap the fruits of your attention and a most broad field of most fascinating things will be disclosed, in which your own thoughts may expand with no less pleasure than utility.

(1a) The "little Frenchman"[1] against whom Gaub's opening remarks were directed was Julien La Mettrie, who was, like Gaub, a physician and a pupil of Hermann Boerhaave, Gaub's great predecessor at Leiden. Gaub's first essay was delivered in the form of a lecture on 8 February 1747, and the publication of *Man a Machine* followed late in the same year.[2] "La Mettrie", Gaub wrote later, "was seated very attentively at the steps of the chair when I spoke this discourse, and a little later he published his man-machine. This made me more cautious with regard to the matter in my Institutions."[3] What made him more cautious was the fact that "certain malicious individuals" had drawn irreligious conclusions from his lecture.[4] He seems to have considered La Mettrie to be the most offensive. While there is no doubt that La Mettrie borrowed certain illustrative material from Gaub's lecture, the material was, so to speak, in the public domain. Furthermore, the initial stimulus to La Mettrie's thoughts along these lines was the same as Gaub's: the great interest in mechanistic explanations of man and the universe characterizing the European intellectual scene from the middle of the seventeenth century on. As for La Mettrie's borrowings they are limited to the following: (a) with reference to the dependency of moral character on bodily temperament he states that Descartes expanded a truth which Galen recognized and adds in a footnote that it was Descartes, not

Hippocrates, as the author of the *Natural History of the Soul* had supposed, who held that the power to change the characters of men for the better would be found in the art of medicine alone; the author of the *Natural History of the Soul* was, of course, La Mettrie himself, and it seems likely that this correction of his own error followed Gaub's lecture,[5] (b) the story of Julius Canus,[6] (c) the instance of pregnancy kleptomania,[7] (d) the bizarre case of pregnancy pica: a wife who killed, salted down and ate her husband piecemeal,[8] (e) the story of Elizabeth of Milan,[9] (f) the cannibal child.[10] These case histories appear in La Mettrie in much the same order as in Gaub. La Mettrie may also have borrowed his remarks on the proper use of food and wine, on the *enormôn*, and on the effects of "bloody foods"[11] from Gaub. We can hardly give La Mettrie credit for putting the Cartesian ideal of the goal of medicine in a new philosophical context with the advantage of a more advanced physiology, as Vartanian claims.[12] Firstly, although the point cannot be argued here, his physiology represents no real advance over that of Descartes, and secondly, the credit (if any is to be given) for elaborating and presenting the "Cartesian ideal" clearly belongs to Gaub. One of the features of Gaub's first lecture, to which La Mettrie listened so intently, was a serious and spirited plea for physicians to engage in a concerted search for corporeal agencies of use in managing the mind. Finally, it must be said that La Mettrie wrote like a pamphleteer rather than a philosopher or scientist and simply ignored the important line of evidence that Gaub gave proper attention (the evidence of immediate experience)—either because he did not grasp its significance or was aware that it conflicted too glaringly with his own oversimplified view of human nature. (1b) We may conveniently inquire into the views of Hermann Boerhaave, the respected teacher of both La Mettrie and Gaub, at this point. The procedure of reasoning *more geometrico*—meaning that a theoretical structure is to be based on a set of axioms from which all other statements are to be derived—had seized his imagination, largely because of its success in mathematical physics.

In the study of medicine he calls for "clear and distinct principles", *à la Descartes*, from which all demonstrations are to be made, but (unlike Descartes) he held that such principles can be founded only on a study of the purely corporeal aspect of man.[13] The first principle of everything that involves figure or motion must be of corporeal nature, and from this principle everything corporeal is to be explained and understood.[14] Boerhaave grants that there is another aspect of man which is neither demonstrable nor explicable on the basis of this principle, since man represents a unity of mind and body and these two entities are of entirely different nature. However, they are joined in such a way that each thought of the mind corresponds to a definite state of the body, although, on the other hand, certain bodily activities take place beyond the awareness and control of the mind. How mind and body can act on one another has not been explained, but observation teaches us that it does occur and this is enough for medicine, a science which finds ultimate metaphysical causes neither available, necessary nor useful.[15] In Boerhaave's definition of disease— any condition limiting the power of the body to exercise any one of its functions, due to the absence of some requisite for or the presence of some hindrance to the exercise of this function—no mention is made of mind because, as he tells us, every mental state is accompanied by a definite bodily state, and the art of medicine can therefore restore the state of the mind by acting on the body.[16] These principles are also discussed by Boerhaave in a well-known lecture given in 1702 in which he sets forth the applicability of mechanistic reasoning in medicine.[17] The "mechanists" are the mathematicians and physicists who have calculated the powers of bodies, reasoning *more geometrico* from mass, figure and velocity. The "clear light of truth" shed by the use of this method has, says Boerhaave, so recommended it to scholars that nothing else that the age has brought forth has been so highly praised and approved. Only in the art of medicine has it been neglected.[18] Yet there is no other key to the understanding of the peculiar structure of the corporeal machine. Either we will find no scientific laws governing here, or the palm will go to the "mechanical method", as far as the understanding and control of the human body is concerned.[19] For the human body is a machine whose solid parts are adapted to the collection, distribution, alteration, separation and secretion of liquids.[20] Those people, he remarks, who claim that the power of mind over body teaches us that life, disease and health depend on some non-mechanical principle, who laugh smugly at what they consider to be vain mechanical speculations, ought instead to deplore our common ignorance. Nevertheless, in spite of this ignorance of the nature of the mind and its relation to the body, all events taking place in the body are corporeal and subject to mechanical law. Whether or not their primary causes are mechanical should not detain us. The mechanistically minded physician need only search out, understand and direct the corporeal effects.[21] (1c) What is meant when these writers call animals or men "machines" is by no means always clear. The term originally signified an instrument, or set of instruments, designed for a specific purpose,[22] and was obviously applicable to the body, with its various arrangements for seizing, biting, holding, moving about, and so forth. To regard the human body (not the human being) as a machine carried with it no taint of impiety (Hamlet, for example, calls himself "this machine" quite naturally—he is no doubt thinking of his "pickers" and "stealers"—and without enunciating a philosophical position; he refers merely to the character of his bodily framework). In the latter part of the seventeenth century we find the pious Boyle attributing crises in disease "to the wisdom and ordinary providence of God, exerting itself by the mechanism partly of that smaller engine the human body".[23] At about the same time Augustin Fasch, professor of anatomy and surgery at Jena, was led to praise the wisdom and kindness of God in regard to that "stupendous machine which is the human body".[24] Mechanism is quite acceptable, it would seem as long as it is (a) not atheistic, (b) limits itself to the corporeal aspect of man, and

(c) does not jeopardize the Christian doctrine of free will. Descartes and La Mettrie, like many others in the seventeenth and eighteenth centuries, have clockwork in mind when they think of machines. Such machines are then *automata*, devices containing their own source of motion (as the original machines did not). Descartes, in fact, says that the body of a living man differs from that of a dead man just as a wound clock differs from one that has run down.[25] The principle of motion in a clock is a bent spring or falling weight, while in men and animals it is some unknown feature of the bodily machinery; Descartes states explicitly—breaking here with tradition—that thought, mind, or soul is *not* this principle of motion in man.[26]   (1d) The most precise and far-reaching definition of mechanism was given by Leibniz in his objections to Georg Stahl's medical system. All truths, Leibniz says, must be derivable from prior truths of the same order, provided that they are not primary. More specifically, every natural event or material state can be derived from knowledge of the preceding event or state, provided that the appropriate laws of change are known as well. This is, Leibniz adds, what those who claim that everything taking place in corporeal bodies is mechanically explicable mean or ought to mean.[27]   (1e) We may turn here to the opinions of some eighteenth-century physicians. Carrère accepts the resemblance of the human body to a machine, but he leaves the motive power of this machine situated, as before, in the mind or soul. The movements of the human body cannot be derived from the arrangement of "these machines" alone. The motive power lies in the *anima*; it is vain to seek for it in the body. In support of his views he cites from Borelli's treatise on animal motion to the effect that the soul is the principle and efficient cause of motion in the bodily machine, i.e. the principle of life and motion in men and animals.[28]   Smith, the medical author of a treatise on the nerves, finds it difficult to understand how anyone can believe that animals are, as the Cartesians claimed, pure machines "framed entirely of matter, so many curious pieces of clockwork, wound up and set a-going". He himself believed that there was a "sentient principle" in animals as well as men.[29] The belief that animals were pure machines had as a corollary the belief that they had no "feelings".[30] Pauli hears Descartes and his "sycophants" crying out that it is absurd to hold that brutes have feelings and emotions. But why else does the dog wag his tail at his master and bite the thief, he demands? Brutes have the same physical equipment as men, and their emotions and emotional disturbances are too obvious to be denied except on the basis of a preconceived opinion.[31] Pauli's reasons of the heart obviously share no common ground with Descartes's reasons of the head. (2a) The personage referred to here was the young prince William V of Orange, who had been placed in Gaub's care by the Estates General in 1760. A panegyric directed at the prince in the closing paragraphs of this lecture has been omitted from the translation. (2b) Gaub, we may recall, stated in the first lecture (§49) that although the action of mind on body was the more important aspect of the relationship between the two, he intended to pass over it for lack of time.

II   The Rational and Irrational Parts of the Mind

4. So that my discussion will follow an orderly course, therefore, I shall first set forth those changes, baneful as well as beneficial, that experience reveals the mind to be capable of exciting in the bodily economy. I shall not be greatly concerned with giving an account of the basis of these changes or explaining the manner of action by which they come about, since I have previously dealt with these matters more fully than should be expected of a physician and I do not blush to admit myself more ignorant now than at that time. If I set forth this group of observations it will then be easy to disclose the safeguards of health offered by the mind in fortune and misfortune.

5. If you yourselves have neither been taught by a certain interior sense nor agree with my previous assertion that the mind contains two very different principles of action, although it seems simple and indivisible in nature, I hope that you will believe Pythagoras and Plato, the wisest of the ancient philosophers, who, according to Cicero, divided the mind into two parts, one partaking of reason and the other devoid of it. In the partaker of reason they placed serenity, that is to say, a calm and quiet steadfastness, in the other those disordered impulses of rage and desire that are the opposites and enemies of reason. And so it is indeed. It should be quite obvious to anyone who attends to what he experiences within himself that some of the mind's activities are temperate, regular, steadfast, of uniform course, coherent and perspicacious; others, on the contrary, are somewhat crude, irregular, inconstant, disconnected, confused and hurried onward by blind impetus. Since they differ so greatly from one another that they seem to fight on opposite fronts, as it were, anyone who believes that they are to be derived from the same active principle will have to attribute opposite effects to one and the same cause. If he does not find it incongruous to assert this he will nevertheless have to admit that the mode of action of the two is very different, and that a mind illuminated by reason is quite unlike itself when disturbed. Since I have already discussed this problem at length, I recall it at this point only so that you will understand the course I have chosen for the treatment of my theme.

(4) Gaub believes that the *philosophical* problem of mind-body interaction is insoluble. His proposed solution of the *physiological* problem is set forth in §§33–44 of the first lecture. (5a) In spite of his claim Gaub is anatomizing the mind in a fashion somewhat different from that of the first lecture. On the former occasion he described the *enormôn*—

the driving force or principle of action—of the mind and its counterpart, the *enormôn* of the body. The corporeal *enormôn*, he then said, is the nervous system itself. One part of it is concerned with sensation and voluntary motion and is in direct communication with the mind. The other part has to do with the natural and vital activities. It is that part of the nervous system, independent of the mind, controlling the involuntary physiological activities. In states of emotional disturbance the mind can affect the latter activities only by virtue of the relation holding between the separate parts of the corporeal *enormôn*. That is to say, in the first lecture Gaub did not divide the *enormôn* of the mind into two parts, as he divided that of the body. But he now suggests that there are *two* principles of action in the mind, which amounts to saying that there are two *enormônta*, one partaking of reason and the other devoid of it. (5b) Plato's division was tripartite actually. To the rational part of the *psychê* he opposed an irrational part, but he divided it into two subdivisions, *thymos* and *epithymia*, one inclining toward, the other away from reason. (5c) Gaub cites the *Tusculan Disputations* of Cicero and quotes him word for word in the passage beginning, "... divided the mind into two parts ..." and ending, "... opposites and enemies of reason ...".[32] Gaub then argues that the differences are so great that the powers of the mind seem to fight on opposite fronts. To derive them from a single active principle would be equivalent to attributing opposite effects to the same cause. He overlooks the solution to this problem offered by Descartes. Descartes argued that the combats supposedly taking place between these two parts of the mind are in reality combats between the mind and the bodily machine. The two wrestle for control at their site of interaction, the pineal gland. Previous writers, he claims, have failed to distinguish the functions of the body from those of the mind. He elaborates this explanation as follows: There are two kinds of movement excited by the "nervous spirits" in the gland. One serves to give the mind a representation of the object that has aroused the senses, the other to arouse the bodily movements which constitute the emotions. Although the first "movement" may interfere with the operations of the mind, or be hindered by them in turn, it does not affect the volition. We are therefore not conscious of a conflict. The second kind of movement does involve a conflict with volition, since a desire may thereby be incited in the mind for something which the mind itself rejects. The mind then feels itself forced, at the same time, to desire and not to desire one and the same thing.[33] Descartes' rejection of the partitioning of the mind is made in such a way as to suggest that everyone before him regarded these partitions as fixed and fast. This is hardly the truth, since the majority of Christian philosophers and theologians, following Augustine, agree that the mind is one. Augustine held that the soul or *anima* is given different names in accordance with its various functions: *anima* when it simply animates or makes alive, *spiritus* when it contemplates, *sensus* when it feels, *animus* when it knows, *mens* when it understands, *ratio* when it discriminates, *memoria* when it records, *voluntas* when it desires—these, he says, are different in name but not in substance. There is only one *anima*.[34]

III   Failure of the Undisturbed Mind to Care Rationally for the Body

6. For although it is rightly believed that the sound, composed mind, using reason as her guide, is so warmly attached to herself and her body that she is obliged to maintain with all zeal and effort the integrity of the body—in the absence of which a feeling of indisposition is unavoidable—and neither permit nor do anything that may disturb the health, it hardly requires to be pointed out that much to the contrary obviously occurs everyday.

7. Indeed!—human reason is not so fortunate as to illuminate the mind in every quarter with the light of certain truth, or to start her off on the right track and at all times keep her from going astray. For man to avoid error in the judgement of a great many matters is difficult, but the difficulty is greatest in those bearing on health and disease, since their number and nature make them very obscure and hard to assess. Given this degree of fallibility of the human spirit it is not remarkable that things happen amiss every day to the detriment of the body in a variety of ways, even when the mind is tranquil. Rare are those who remain untouched.

8. Time would fail me were I to review and give instances of the countless errors committed. I shall not recall how frequently the offense comes from pitiful ignorance and how many there are who have at one time or another been led astray by a desire for novelty, the customs of the times or the unwise imitation of others, by a misplaced faith in their own powers and the deceptive safeguard of habit, by the impunity hoped for because the penalty was delayed and by inexcusable carelessness, so that they provide for the mind neither by preserving the healthy climate in which it flourishes nor by obtaining the needful when health fails. In a thousand ways a matter whose importance exceeds my powers of expression is made into a plaything. This fault is common to men of every condition, and one may rightfully regret that the instinct of brute beasts is often less unreasonable than reason is in us.

9. There I see the philosopher spending the whole day in his musty study, neglecting bodily exercise, so agape in the consumption of books that he will not grant an hour of a sunny summer day to a stroll in which his foul lungs may be refreshed by the use of fresh air. For my part you may warn, beseech, chide and importune him; you will be deceived and in the

end will unhappily fall silent as you see the sage forced into immobility—his chest filled with phlegm, his joints rigid, his feet swollen with watery fluid and incapable of motion. A glorious thing it is, of course, to die prematurely for the sake of wisdom!

10. Contrast him now, gentlemen, with another man of iron constitution, who rejoices in a strong body and bountiful health and, lest he seem to disregard his bounties, makes free with them by vigorously indulging his appetites. Indeed there is nothing in the way of food, drink, climate, lack of sleep, exertion and so forth that he cannot bear with impunity. He, too, laughs at the physician who dares to urge moderation, unaware that many blows may break that which one cannot and persuading himself with doltish arguments that he will not be harmed tomorrow or at any future time by whatever did not harm him yesterday or the day before. Oh unbelievable folly! Oh judgement, less to be healed by three Anticyras than by one's own experience of a premature death!

11. Would that this kind of man made a fool of himself alone! But we see that he sets a bad example for others to follow. By no means everyone can assess himself with his own rule and measure. Hence it is that those who are weaker by nature consider that they too are likewise free to do without harm what they see done and borne with impunity by their companions. Even when frightened by the harmful effects they do not leave off in time, relying on the vain hope that their constitutions will become toughened by use. Constantly struggling between crime and punishment these unfortunates, like the Phrygians, finally become wise too late.

12. No less is the madness of those who, their eyes fixed on the same examples, become far too conscious of how much weaker they are, and would prefer to be more like these others than like themselves. Averse to the foolhardiness of the first group, yet discontented

with their own powers, they fall therefore into the opposite error and put all hope of improving their health in the continual use of remedies. As if differences in degree of health of the body, like differences of the human face, were not limited by fixed natural laws, as if physicians could at will make all alike! An erroneous opinion! Not only do those who hold it miss their aim, many of them die before their time as well, their natural powers weakened by the abuse of medicaments. They deserve the epitaph—untranslatable into Latin—*stavo ben, ma per star meglio, sto qui,* said to stand on tombs in Italy.

13. Do you require other examples, gentlemen? Shall I speak of the harm that tender young girls, pregnant women and handsome youths inflict on their bodies when they allow themselves to be urged on by the breath of light spirits to neglect their health and contrive a whole mode of life completely dependent on the changing fashions of the times, to make daily alterations in dress, ornaments, food, social intercourse and amusements that are rarely more in keeping with moderation than over-indulgence? Shall I touch on the precautionary measures based solely on custom and practiced indiscriminately by many people in the spring and autumn, measures that far more frequently provoke rather than protect the health? Shall I lament the dull credulity of those who mistrust nature and the art that is her minister, but are ready to entrust life and health—which ought to be man's most precious possessions—to windy quacks, nostrum venders and barber surgeons, nay more, to trust their heads to wretched cobblers whom no one would allow to fit shoes on his feet? But I am ashamed to make public more such reproaches to the human reason of this kind. They can hardly please your ears, since recollection of similar stupidities perpetrated by each of us at one time or another will come to mind and trouble us with secret shame.

(6) It is a Christian belief, or at least part of the Christian tradition, that the mind loves the body in somewhat the same sense that God loves the world. It follows, perhaps, from the analogy often drawn between the two, the mind or soul standing in more or less the same relationship (although with certain definite restrictions) to the material framework of the body that God does to the universe, i.e. God is the "soul of the world". (7) In stressing the fallibility of the human spirit, as he does here, Gaub is perfectly orthodox. (8) Later on (§31) Gaub states that instinct is quasi-rational. Here he contrasts it with reason, and points out that animals may derive more benefit from this source than we ourselves do from the light of reason.[35] (9) See Gaub I, §54 and commentary, where the dangerous effects of overstraining the mind and neglecting the body are discussed. (10a) The man of iron constitution[36] abuses the non-naturals with impunity. His reasoning, too, is faulty, since there are limits to every man's powers. (10b) Anticyra was the source of hellebore, a purgative and emetic used in the treatment of insanity by the Greeks and Romans. There were three towns of that name, in Locris Ozolis, Malis and Phocis, but the last-named, lying on the Corinthian Gulf, seems to have been the chief source.[37] (11) As in the previous essay Gaub emphasizes the variability of individual men in response to the same harmful agencies. The Phrygians, to whom the unfortunates who become wise too late are compared, were proverbial among the Greeks and Romans for their stupidity. (12) The epitaph here represents a play on the meanings of the verb *"stare"* in Italian, and is not readily translatable into English. *"Stare ben"* is to be comfortable enough, *"stare qui"* is to rest here. Gerard van Swieten quotes the same proverb in commenting on the baneful effects of excessive bleeding and purging on patients.[38] (13a) A study of the maladies of the fashionable world of the eighteenth century was written by Simon-André Tissot.[39] He remarks that physicians have composed books on diseases of the poor, diseases of workers, and diseases of sailors, and he himself was the

author of a book on diseases of the court; only the diseases of *gens du monde* have been neglected.[40] The peculiarity of these people, from the medical standpoint, lies in their desire to be cured while continuing to espouse a way of life which will inevitably ruin their health. They eat too much, drink excessively, turn night into day, and spend too much time indoors.[41] The women wear constricting clothing that harms their internal organs and interferes with breathing and digestion.[42] We smile at the Chinese whose women deform their feet with bandages, yet we ourselves force young girls to pass much of their lives in whalebone vises that not only prevent proper growth and interfere with vital functions but make them suffer abominably as well.[43] Our women cover their heads with resins that block transpiration and smear their faces with pomades containing harmful agents such as mercury and lead.[44] Both men and women of this class are far more subject to emotional disturbances giving rise to harmful effects in the body than are peasants.[45] (13b) The phrase "nature and the art that is her minister" is an indication of Gaub's Hippocratism. The physician is the minister of nature, as he writes elsewhere, in accordance with the Hippocratic dictum that nature is the true physician of disease.[46]

IV Emotional Disturbances and Personal Responsibility

14. I pass on, in accordance with my plan, to the disturbed mind. Acquiring a far more unrestrained and unlawful power over the body it is then, as might readily be supposed, so much the more able to inflict even worse bodily ills. Of these I can speak more freely, however, since they have the excuse of weakness—if not a lawful excuse yet one that it seems possible to approve—and hence merit more pity than scorn.

15. I freely admit that the philosophers are right in requiring the mind to check her own *enormôn* with the

reins of right reason, thus mitigating its force and preventing it from breaking out of bounds. Yet how many persons, I ask, are calm and steadfast enough not to be overwhelmed at some time by the unbelievable number of chance accidents to which we are continually exposed? How often do errors in perception, figments of the imagination and mistakes in judgement mislead mortal man? I believe that in my first lecture I have more than sufficiently shown how the body itself, in consequence of age, sex, temperament, disease and mode of life, acts rapidly and violently on its parts, and how the unwilling and struggling mind is often overthrown from its state, as everyday experience shows. Were I now to plead the cause of the mind it would be easy for me to cite much that would diminish or excuse her guilt. However, I feel that I am obliged to recount rather those baneful effects which the body suffers from the mind. Yet I am uncertain just how to accomplish this in an orderly and fitting way. So numerous and different in character are they that there is indeed no manner of disease or death that may not flow from this source, and he who would wish to recount each and every one would be forced to present almost the whole of medical nosology.

(14) Gaub means that while the human being cannot refuse responsibility for his acts on the ground of a "disturbed mind"[47] we can nevertheless admit this as a mitigating circumstance. Here he is referring mainly to the effects of strong emotions on the behavior. (15a) The phrase "right reason"[48] is one of Cicero's favorites, and it appears in the *Tusculan Disputations* in the paragraph following the one cited by Gaub in §5. In this passage Cicero calls strong emotions disturbances of the mind "opposed to right reason". Where Gaub says that irrational impetus of the mind should be kept in check by right reason (although the influence of various corporeal factors sometimes makes this an impossible task) Cicero says that an emotionally

disturbed mind can no more check its headlong rush than a
criminal flung from the promontory of Leucas his fall.⁴⁹
(15b) Descartes ascribed to the mind absolute power to
control the actions of the body and thus to check the movements incited in it by the passions, with reference, of course,
only to those movements normally under the control of the
will.   Man cannot control his passions, using this word in
its broadest signification, but he can control his actions.
The will is free by nature, Descartes writes, thus subscribing
to Christian doctrine.⁵⁰

V   External and Internal Changes in the Body
Produced by the Emotions

16. I gladly omit whatever the mind perpetrates at
times to the detriment of the bodily economy and the
endangerment of life itself when struggling under some
affliction of the body, confused by the weakness of its
organs or aroused by the violence of feverish movements and rendered desperate by insufferable pain and
anguish.   It is fitting that these, originating primarily
in the body, be reckoned also to its account.   I wish
to speak of those which a mind disturbed by her own
impetus brings about when her thoughts tend toward
the good or bad believed to lie under the surface of
things and she conceives desires or aversions that are
adhered to more violently and tenaciously than is
warranted.   Are any of you unaware, gentlemen, of
the extent to which a disturbed mind can affect the
outward appearance of the body?   Of the manner in
which different affections, whatever their nature, lead
to one kind of change or another in the face, eyes,
forehead and the other outward parts, each one
picturing itself abroad with its own peculiar characteristics, so that there is no need to wish for a little window
in the breast to observe what the unquiet mind con-
ceals beneath?   If they erupt to the surface in such

number and profusion think how much more violently the interior parts where they arise must be disturbed, since these parts have far less power of resistance and perform as well services for the welfare of the economy that are in fact much more important.

(16) Gaub states that he will not consider those disturbances arising secondarily in the mind as a result of bodily disease and then reacting on the body to produce further harm. He will limit himself to the bodily effects of disturbances arising primarily in the mind, that is, to the effects of the emotions.[51] After calling attention, as in the first lecture (§27), to the outward changes brought on by strong emotions he suggests that the less resistant internal organs may suffer even more severely. Similar remarks can be found in Cicero, Seneca and Celsus,[52] and the external manifestations of the emotions are often described minutely, as we shall see, in seventeenth- and eighteenth-century medical literature. Descartes, too, devotes considerable attention to these changes, and notes that every emotion is revealed by a characteristic action of the eyes—even the most stupid servant, he says, can tell from the eyes of his master whether he is in or out of favor.[53]

VI Harmful Effects of Acute Anger on the Body

17. I shudder to recall the damage, seen with my own eyes or heard of by word of mouth, inflicted on the body by an irate mind. In one man swelling anger rages in the lower viscera and vomiting, diarrhea, bile and jaundice set everything in disorder. In another, the most deadly, burning, inflammatory, putrid, eruptive and malignant fevers result, as the disturbance breaks out in the circuit of the blood. If its force is directed within an incurable dilatation of the heart occurs. At another time the special workshop of the

mind is not spared.   Nor does anger always explode as a brief madness, for it sometimes throws the organs of sense and motion into convulsions, delirium, madness, paralysis and apoplexy, marring them with irremediable defects.   These terrible things happen even to the strongest of men.   How much more that is dreadful may happen to the weak and the ailing, to those who are afflicted by disease or convalescing from illness, whenever a violent flare-up occurs!   Let the feverish, the gouty, the epileptic, the colicky, the asthmatic, those affected with stone, the hysterical, the pregnant and the post-partum be witness that when anger swells the disease under which they labor most often grows worse and is aggravated by new attacks or changes from mild to malignant.   The attacks are hastened, the greatly hoped-for aids of nature and the art are subverted, and death instead of recovery is the outcome.   The most trivial injuries are thus at times fatal, and capital punishment would be imposed on the assailant did not the expert judgement of our gracious faculty intervene.

18. You will rightly marvel, gentlemen, at the enormous number of afflictions that anger alone, as if from Pandora's box, spreads abroad in the body.   It is not difficult to discover the source of all the mischief. Beyond what is clearly established—that the motive powers distributed throughout the organs of the body are greatly aroused by this paroxysm of the mind, and that the entire framework, including all of the viscera, vessels and humors contained within, is shaken by violent movements—something that almost passes belief is plain from numerous observations, namely, that the natural properties of the humors are so greatly altered as to corrupt them with incredible speed from mild to acrid, from healthful to harmful or even poisonous.   Do you doubt this?   I cite an hysterical woman who vomited corrupted bile of all colors and degrees of acridity when attacked by her illness in a

fit of rage, an angry nurse whose breasts instilled in place of nutriment a deadly poison into her suckling with frightful convulsions, tamed and domestic animals who become rabid when provoked and discharge the poison in their foaming saliva into men whom they bite, and the case of a man bitten by one of two Gallic cocks on intervening between them when they were furiously fighting, as is their custom, who died of hydrophobia rising from the wound. You will perhaps plead the difference between man and beast, hence I shall offer in addition instances from our own kind. A soldier was brawling with a woman who bit and wounded his hand. The man was seized by a rigor and died. A furiously angered Italian youth who was unable to revenge himself gnawed at his own finger and was carried away by fatal hydrophobia, just as if he had been bitten by a rabid dog. I am well aware and readily admit that I do not understand how the poisonous corruption of the humors so quickly comes about. Nevertheless, I have made you understand, I believe, that the universal foundation of life is convulsed by this emotion and consequently that there is no function of the human economy able to face such a tumult intact.

(17a) Gaub summarizes here the changes ascribed to acute anger by physicians of his day. In his textbook he states further that anger excites the nerves and muscles, and thereby the movement of the blood and bile, in this way bringing about fever, inflammation and digestive disturbances.[54] We recall from the first lecture that an emotion is said to begin as a disturbance of the mind based on a judgement, to spread to the voluntary nervous system, and finally to arouse the involuntary nervous system, i.e. that part of the nervous system controlling the "natural and vital functions".[55] Not only the visceral organs controlled by the nervous system but the nervous system itself, specifically the brain, the "special workshop of the mind", may suffer damage as a result of the circulatory disturbance, Gaub tells us. (17b) Anger is not always a "brief madness" (the classic definition of Horace) since it may produce lasting irremediable damage in the healthy and aggravate the diseases of the ill.[56] The last sentence of the paragraph evidently means that expert witnesses from the medical faculty had on occasion testified that deaths apparently due to physical assault were actually due to the corporeal effects of anger induced by the assault.[57] (17c) It should be understood that Gaub was merely repeating the generally accepted medical opinion of his time in making these claims, as the following will show. We turn first to Boerhaave, who says that when a man succumbs to anger there is room in him for little else. There is a faculty or power inherent in man activated in emotional disturbances and capable of giving rise to all of the changes ordinarily incited by corporeal causes. As if imbued with heat, the angry man swells, tremors shake his limbs and, if the disturbance is sufficiently great, his blood itself grows thicker. Everything about him is changed—his voice sticks in his throat, he breathes deeply, his heart palpitates and he may lose consciousness. Nausea, vomiting, loss of appetite, diarrhea, rumbling of the bowels, griping colic, flatus, and a flow of urine may occur all against his will. And in this way, Boerhaave adds, troubling diseases may arise.[58] Anger readies the body for revenge, according to Pechlin. The humors and spirits boil up, the solid parts of the body are as if inflated, and the full strength of its members set free.[59] Tremors, irregularities of heart action, and epileptiform convulsions may occur when anger is severe.[60] Zückert says that in the grip of anger man frequently loses all control over himself. Running madly about he stamps his feet, grinds his teeth, strikes his fist on the table, snorts, fumes and foams at the mouth, utters the most frightful curses, conjures up all the furies, all the devils of hell, to help his revenge and threatens his enemy with fire, sword and murder. Everything in his path becomes the object of his wrath. He hurls chairs, benches and tables about. In the face of his fury wife, child, maid and man, friend and foe must fly. The unhappy offender who falls into his hands is treated in a barbaric fashion. Glasses are thrown at his head, he is knocked to the floor, trampled on, and dragged about by the hair. Apoplexy, bilious fever, bilious colic, and consumption can result, Zückert claims, from excessive anger.[61] Corp finds that anger increases the rate of circulation and respiration and may cause hemorrhages from the nose, ears, lungs, anus and uterus. More important effects, including paralysis, apoplexy, and sudden death, may occur in persons of advanced age and sanguine temperament. The influence of anger over the organs of respiration is only equalled by its effects on the secretion of bile, and it is for this reason that an episode of anger is often followed by a profuse evacuation of bile. This has led some to believe that a superabundance, or some other such disturbance, of the bile is the cause of anger. Persons afflicted with jaundice due to gall-stones should avoid attacks of this emotion. Such concretions, Corp says, may remain in the gall-bladder for many years without causing jaundice, but it may occur if they are shifted in position so as to obstruct the passage of bile into the intestine. Bodily exertion is likely to have this effect, and since anger agitates the entire framework of the body, Corp adds, it may cause jaundice.[62] Laroque describes the suffused face, glittering eye, foaming lips and convulsive movements of the angry man, and mentions apoplexy, paralysis, jaundice, rupture of blood-vessels in the lungs, hemorrhage and sudden death as consequences.[63] Jaundice is the subject of Morgagni's 37th letter, and although he does not specifically mention anger as a factor in any of his cases his remarks are of interest since he does discuss jaundice due to emotional disturbances. After presenting one instance of fatal jaundice following "a kind of perturbation of mind", with rather indefinite autopsy findings, he remarks that the effects of emotions in bringing on jaundice has been confirmed by numerous medical observations, nor should this be surprising when we consider how the "nerves consent with the passions, and the power of these same nerves over the blood and excretory vessels and consequently in impeding and vitiating the secretions and excretions of the humors". If we suppose that the hepatic nerves consent most or yield most easily to the action of the nerves, jaundice from "passions of the mind" is easy, he says, to understand.[64] In another of Morgagni's patients, who was terrified by a ruffian who threatened to shoot him, jaundice and delirium appeared on the following day, and he died twenty-four hours thereafter. Nothing of note was observed at autopsy. Morgagni regards the case as one of jaundice due to fright brought on by "contraction of the hepatic nerves".[65] (18a) The motive powers Gaub refers to here lie within the control of the corporeal *enormôn*, the driving force of the nervous system. Specifically, he means the powers controlling digestion, respiration and other natural and vital, that is, physiological, functions. The natural healing powers, including inflammation, fever, and many other automatic "movements" leading to the expulsion of noxious matter from the body are included.[66] (18b) Gaub's claim that anger can bring about alterations in the chemical composition of the body fluids may be found in his textbook as well.[67] He regards hydrophobia as the consequence of a poisonous alteration of the body fluids brought on by extreme rage. Although he gives no source he is probably drawing from a case report by J. B. Scaramucci, published in 1702.[68] The patient, a youth of twenty years with a choleric temperament, became febrile an unspecified time after biting himself, then averse to water, mad and uncontrollable; he died a short time afterward. Scaramucci regarded this as an instance of true hydrophobia. To support his claim that the disease need not be due to the bite of a mad dog or cat he brings forward a case of hydrophobia from the bite of a fighting cock, evidently the one mentioned by Gaub. His explanation is as follows: a disturbance of the nervous spirits alters the humors of the body so as to produce a poison which is then transmitted by the bite. He adds that anger is a brief madness, according to Seneca, and hydrophobia itself is a kind of madness.[69]

(18c) Boerhaave ascribes changes in the humors brought about by the emotions to the power of the common sensorium, the power that Paracelsus called the imagination, Hippocrates the *impetum faciens* and others the *anima*.[70] I have seen, Boerhaave tells us, a healthy woman, with a healthy nursing infant at her breast, who became involved in a brawl and grew angry and excited while she continued to nurse her child. Within a short time the child developed convulsions. Who knows, he asks, how the change was brought about and what the substance appearing in the milk could have been? Prudence, however, requires us to keep an infant from the breast of an emotionally disturbed nurse. It is understandable, he writes, that an inebriated nurse will make the infant drunk, but it is not easy to see how milk can be so changed by an effect of the mind alone.[71] According to Corp, too, anger is capable of inducing changes in the fluids of the body. He does not believe that an infant can imbibe the virtues or disposition of the person who suckles it, but he has no doubt that milk may be rendered harmful by the operation of anger or other strong emotions. All who give suck should therefore preserve a well-regulated frame of mind. Corp adds that anger is especially dangerous for pregnant women, since not only uterine hemorrhages but fatal miscarriages may result.[72]

VII Harmful Effects of Suppressed Anger on the Body

19. This being so, I am now of the opinion, gentlemen, that all of you will fervently wish and secretly resolve to control yourselves in the future, whatever the occasion for anger may be, for the sake of your health. A wise and praiseworthy intent, yet one not invariably of benefit to everyone! I cannot, indeed, conceal from you the fact that even repressed anger is not always without its bad effects. As a fermenting new wine to which no vent is given damages the cask,

so a raging mind that reason tries to control but cannot calm attacks the body the more violently within to the extent that it is not allowed to discharge itself without. I have mourned, and still mourn, the calamitous death, hastened by no other cause, of a man celebrated throughout the world for his character and accomplishments—a man to whom vigorous bodily strength, a moderate course throughout all of life's stages, and the wishes of the public gave hope of Nestorian years. Doubtless irascible by nature, he had learned from the study of philosphy to repress his anger, but when wounded one day by an unexpected and severe affront, although he did indeed contain his rage, he was so deeply and badly shaken within that he could not escape an early death brought on by a defect arising in his vital parts. I could say more, but I see that the wealth of material has led me to spend a greater time on one emotion than is fitting.

(19) The comparison of repressed anger seeking an outlet to new wine without a vent can be found in the Old Testament.[73] Gaub's claim that anger is capable of damaging the internal organs when denied its normal outlet is more specific but by no means original, although many eighteenth-century writers on the subject of the emotions fail to make it. Georg Stahl claims to have seen men who were overcome by fatal fevers after suppressing their anger, and there are many earlier reports of the same general nature.[74]

VIII   Harmful Effects of Grief on the Body

20. And so I pass on to sorrow. No one is unaware that when it is not discharged in lamentation and wailing, but instead remains seated firmly within and is for a long time repressed and fostered, the body no less than the mind is eaten up and destroyed. The motive powers of the whole bodily economy grow fatigued with continual mourning, the innate strength

of the solid parts decreases, the vital, natural and animal movements become sluggish, whence follow slower circulation of the blood, atrabiliary condensation and pungency of the humors, loss of appetite, indigestion, anorexia, obstruction of the viscera, jaundice, scirrhus, dropsy, melancholy, feeble-mindedness, palsy, catalepsy, lethargy and death. I find that the instances of Endymion's sleep set forth in medical history, of sleep prolonged for months or years are, provided that they are not unworthy of belief, due to grief alone. Since sense and not life is lost, the duration rather than the danger of such episodes excites fear. It is of graver import that sorrow is known to be associated with sudden death. Do I dare call on Niobe and the Heliades as witnesses —the one changed into a rock by sorrow, the others into trees? Who will hold that there is not truth in the stories of the poets? But I prefer to omit the doubtful when I have at hand the certain.

21. Take just one from the memoirs of Michael Montaigne. When King Ferdinand was waging war against the widow of King John of Hungary, one of the mailed knights, his identity hidden beneath an iron casque, performed brilliantly in a certain battle near the town of Buda. Pierced by a spear, he fell at last, after having attracted general attention with his unusual bravery and endurance. All praised and mourned the distinguished warrior, and after the battle was over they sought to find out just who he was. A noble German named Raisciac, greatly moved by this unusual instance of heroism, was standing by the corpse when the casque was lifted and recognized the body as that of his own son. The lamenting bystanders gave utterance to their grief in words and tears; he alone was silent, his dry eyes fixed in stupefaction on the body of his son; he grew rigid, suddenly fell to the ground, and breathed his last. A similar and more recent instance comes to mind that many of you, gentlemen, will at

once recall when I touch upon it. A certain friend of mine, a man highly esteemed in this city, was shocked by the report of the unexpected death of his brother. He at once rented a coach and hurried to the mortuary in The Hague. He saw the departed and was stupefied; he sat down, grew faint, and slipped lifeless from the chair; he was borne to the tomb together with his brother in the same funeral procession. The sorrowing mind withdraws into itself and suspends the flow of the vital humors of the body to such a degree that the blood accumulates in the heart and lungs, and imminent suffocation and death threaten.

(20a) Sorrow, too, if not discharged outwardly will express itself inwardly to the detriment of both mind and body. The sequence of change described here moves, in modern terminology, from the functional to the structural or organic. Atrabiliary condensation and pungency,[75] in the context of Gaub's humoral pathology, means that a loss of water increases the coherence of the solid constituents of the humors; this favors interference with flow through the various channels of the body, hence stagnation and obstruction result and the normally bland humors then become acrid or pungent.[76] (20b) Endymion's sleep, which derives its name from the love of the moon-goddess, Selene, for the shepherd Endymion, is not mentioned by Gaub's contemporaries as a consequence of grief.[77] (20c) Niobe, wife of the king of Thebes, whose seven sons and seven daughters were killed by Apollo and Artemis, was perhaps not "all tears", as Hamlet claims; her difficulty was, rather, that she did not discharge her sorrow in lamentations and wailings, to borrow Gaub's words. In the next paragraph Gaub cites Montaigne as the source of his second instance of overwhelming grief, and in the same chapter Montaigne mentions the story of Niobe as an allegory of the numbing effect of great sorrow.[78] (20c) Zückert, too, warns against the suppression of the outward manifestations of grief. Tears not only relieve the sufferer but have beneficial corporeal effects in addition, since the alternate expansion and contraction of the lungs favors the passage of blood through their vascular channels. Nor is there any disgrace in tears, for strong men as well as weaklings shed them— not only tears of sorrow but of regret, sympathy, joy and anger. Sorrow may engender diseases that are worse, says Zückert, than its original occasion; when it is improperly borne the natural forces of the body are weakened at their source, the action of the heart grows feeble, the humors swell and their passage is blocked.[79] Corp lists nausea, insomnia, emaciation, weakening of the circulation, congestion and obstruction of the abdominal viscera among the effects of severe or protracted grief, one of whose frequent causes is homesickness.[80] Smith says that acute severe grief may cause hysterical convulsions, while long-continued grief will weaken the tone of the stomach, destroy the appetite, interfere with digestion and impair memory and judgement.[81] Numerous observations of the same kind are made by older writers.[82] (21) Gaub's explanation of the cause of sudden death in grief is not altogether implausible and, assuming the occurrence of a similar event in our colder time, a modern pathologist might have little better to offer.

IX Harmful Corporeal Effects of Terror

22. I willingly pass over the similar ills brought about by fear, envy and hatred, lest I annoy you with frequent repetition or seem to want to exaggerate the already sufficiently grave faults of the mind.

23. Terror, the most violent of the emotions, remains. Instances of its fatal effects are everywhere to be seen, nor should this surprise anyone, as its occasions are almost unavoidable in common life and its sudden attack anticipates even the most ready judgement. I would cite those available, as numerous as they are striking, did not the daily conversation of men, in which hardly any other cause of disease or

death is spoken of more frequently than terror, make this idle. Its baneful effects are so numerous and their severity so incredible because it attacks from all quarters armed with all weapons, so to speak, while each of the other emotions causes damage in some one characteristic fashion. I would seem to abuse your patience, gentlemen, were I to wish to set forth in detail at this point the frequency and severity of the affections often caused by those empty yet frightening bugbears that boys commonly make merry with in play and thoughtless females use without hesitation to pacify children, were I to recall the pains, anxieties, losses of voice, fainting spells, cramps, tremors, convulsions, fits, catalepsies, strokes, paralyses, madnesses of various kinds and sudden deaths so often recorded in the memory of every era as results of terror in strong healthy adults—and how much more frequently in persons enfeebled by age, overly delicate due to sex, temperament and way of life, or weakened by disease! —were I to mention the men renowned in our art who are moved by the weight of observation to hold that the origin of pestilences and the like spread by contagion ought especially to be attributed to terror and fear, were I to recall the abundance of uterine fruit—I shall say nothing of what is cut off by abortion, since this is a trifle and familiar enough—disfigured by birthmarks, blemishes and all manner of weaknesses, harassed by wounds, mutilated, maimed, headless and removed in a thousand ways from humankind, whose woes are due to the tremendous power of action— attested to by innumerable stories among the common people and not regarded as incredible by some distinguished minds—lent by terror to the imaginations of pregnant women.

(22) Fear (*metus*) is considered here to be a milder form of terror (*terror*), which is dealt with in the next paragraph. Elsewhere Gaub says that fear may lead to loss of muscle

power, loosening of the sphincters, suppression of perspiration, pallor and trembling, while envy and hatred may cause insomnia, low-grade fever, loss of appetite and emaciation.[83] (23a) Gaub's catalogue of the baneful effects of terror is almost endless.[84] Although he seems here to share, together with many of his contemporaries, the belief that strong emotions in the mother can adversely affect the fetus, he does not mention it in his textbook. There he remarks only that by acting on the nervous system so as to produce contraction of small blood-vessels, hence cramps and convulsions, terror may induce abortion.[85] (23b) Stahl mentions terror as a cause of epileptic attacks in children, and described the case of a woman who became jaundiced from fear of her husband. He suggests that deeply rooted fear may increase susceptibility to plague.[86] Holland notes that some "distinguished physiologists" have attempted to differentiate fear[87] from terror[88] as depressive and excitatory emotions, respectively. He considers this distinction untenable and regards terror as an extreme degree of fear, usually of sudden onset. In fear, he remarks, the powers of sexual embrace may be lost. Terror is reported to have caused convulsions, epilepsy, abortion, violent fever and sudden death.[89] Gaub's misgivings regarding the use of bugbears are shared by Zückert who says that the frightful pictures imprinted in the minds of children are a later source of fear and terror.[90] Corp is even more emphatic. Fear is a debilitating passion, and a disposition to succumb to it may be acquired from the circumstances of one's early life. Every parent should therefore guard against the narration of "those silly and terrific stories" which haunt the nursery. They may render the nervous system liable in the future to be strongly affected by trivial causes.[91] He states that every medical practitioner is well aware of the unfavorable effects of fear, citing a relevant observation of his own in an athletic man of forty whose leg had to be amputated above the knee. All went well except for the patient's extreme fear of death and firm conviction that he was about to die. For no apparent reason, says Corp, he wasted away and expired.[92]   Corp also regards terror as the extremity of fear; it may be accompanied by palpitation and suspension of heart action, irregular respiration, cold skin, sweating and loss of voice.   One of his patients, a woman who had been badly frightened by a burglar, was found apparently lifeless in bed, her pulse weak and her face and extremities cold. Later she developed intermittent fever and recovered only after a long period of debility.[93]   The increased susceptibility to contagious disease as a result of emotional disturbance mentioned by Gaub is described also by Corp, who states that those "whose minds are depressed by fear" are most frequently attacked when epidemic or contagious disorders prevail in England.   Corp had observed that when someone inadvertently entered a house where a patient lay ill with smallpox he would often "immediately sicken" on being apprised of the fact, although he had unknowingly borne the exposure with impunity in the past.[94]   Juncker offers an explanation for such observations.   Those who are seized by terror feel a sensation in the skin as of coldness and bristling due to spastic contraction of its fibers.   Transpiration is thus suppressed and, presumably (although he is not explicit here) the natural defences against disease are weakened.[95]   Valangin, too, agrees that fear may increase susceptibility to contagious diseases.   "Those who were most afraid of the plague were soonest taken with it" he writes, quoting Diemerbroeck, however, rather than describing his own experience.[96]   He mentions also a man who was sentenced to be beheaded.   The sentence was mitigated without telling the prisoner; he was merely struck in the back of the neck with a twig yet he expired at once on receiving the blow.[97]   Pechlin says that fear, timidity and grief encourage the onset of many diseases and he calls it a common observation that this occurs in plague.   His explanation is that the lessened resistance of the timid and sorrowful attracts the poison of plague which pervades the air.   This "lessened resistance" is due to a decrease in the force of the elastic fluids of the body that makes it easier for the contagion to obtain entrance and, once admitted, more difficult to expel. Pechlin suggests that fear and sorrow may have something to do with both the onset and the recurrence, after surgical removal, of cancer of the breast.[98] In general, he holds, fear may arouse or worsen disease. Nothing is more dangerous when disease is abroad than to occupy oneself with fearful or sad ideas, since nothing is easier than for these ideas to be transferred into the body. It seems probable, he says, that when the animal spirits are thus busied with sad thoughts some change is brought about in the closely related vital spirits and thereby transmitted to the blood. Pechlin repeats the claim that in epidemic diseases the fearful are the first affected, and adds that he has seen people who were brought into the presence of the pest become convinced that they themselves were affected to the point that their fear ingeniously counterfeited the symptoms of the disease. Certain of them passed from fear of the disease to the disease itself and finally to death.[99] He witnessed with his own eyes, he tells us, many cases of disease and death brought on by sheer terror when the Frenchman raged through Batavia with fire and sword eighteen years ago.[100] A singular symptom of extreme fear, Pechlin remarks, is rapid greying of the hair. It is rare in young men, but he has seen a youth of twenty who suffered shipwreck and lived for three days in constant fear of death; the hair of his head turned from black to white in this short time.[101] Of the physiological effects of fear Pechlin mentions diarrhea and urgency.[102] Holland, too, states that the sphincters may relax,[103] as do Corp,[104] Smith,[105] Mercer[106] and Valangin,[107] Corp pointing out that this is a common phenomenon in recruits when the prospect of immediate action presents itself, and that animals may be similarly affected. Boerhaave describes the extraordinary case of a man in financial difficulties who, on receiving notice that his lands were to be sold to settle his debts, was so struck by terror and anxiety that he discharged seminal fluid.[108] Mercer[109] and Holland[110] say that fear may suppress lactation. Holland[111] and Laroque[112] say that it may suppress menstruation as well.

X   Emotions Aroused by Anticipated Good May Have Harmful Corporeal Effects

24. Although I have omitted much and touched lightly on details in passing, I am well aware that I have been far too circumstantial, yet I must nevertheless hold you to this topic for a little while longer. For you may perhaps believe that only the kind of emotion induced by the gloomy thought of approaching evil rages through the mind with the violence that I have described, whereas when we are aroused and attracted by the happy picture of anticipated good whatever force surges up is not harmful at all but is rather of benefit to both parties. Since the facts are quite otherwise I hope, gentlemen, that you will permit me to mention in passing some common instances from which you will understand that emotions of this other kind may, when they flare up violently, oppress the bodily economy with harshness, equal force and twin tyranny.

25. Not to digress further I shall say nothing of the baneful effects of extravagant laughter, the companion of foolishly unrestrained joy, which often causes bloody sputum, pleurisy, peripneumonia, loss of sense and even sudden death when it breaks out in violent tumults. Nor shall I recall the heavy but not undeserved punishment of those who, carried away by the blind fury of unbridled lust and following their various urges, are hurried into every kind of voluptuousness only to tire out at last, their natural powers shattered by an unrestrained mode of life. Even if these are due primarily to intemperance of the mind they nevertheless admit secondary and less remote causes deriving from pre-existing bodily weakness. I shall give some more important and appropriate examples of what the heated and excited mind effects in the pith and marrow of the body with her own proper impetus.

(24) According to the Stoic philosophy emotional disturbances are to be avoided under all circumstances, whether or not the object occasioning them is regarded as good or bad. Gaub will later state (§48) that he is not in favor of inculcating the apathy of the Stoics into his patients. This follows from the doctrine of the non-naturals, of course, which holds that the emotions may at times have beneficial effects on the body and that the effect is largely independent of the type of emotion concerned. (25) The effects of unbridled lust (which is a desire for something thought good) are indirect and remote, hence not to the point. Gaub claims, too, that there are secondary causes in the body responsible for the behavior of libertines, even though the primary cause is intemperance of the mind.[113] Gaub's phraseology here suggests that he was again consulting Cicero, since he speaks of what the "heated and excited mind effects in the pith and marrow of the body".[114] Cicero, in a discussion of the validity of the Stoic analogy of diseases of the body and diseases of the mind, states that when the disturbed condition of the mind becomes fixed, then it takes root, so to speak, in the pith and marrow as a disease.[115] In this passage Cicero does not mean, as Gaub does, that the body becomes diseased in the face of long-standing emotional disturbance, but rather that such a disturbance constitutes disease of the mind.

XI   Harmful Corporeal Effects of Unrequited Love

26. How the force and continuity of the functions slacken, how the condition of the body languishes and all powers of the economy weaken and collapse when an ardent wish for some desired object is too long drawn out! Do not even the sturdiest races exhibit men who are troubled by peculiar ailments when assailed by a yearning, to which they do not yield soon enough, to return home after having tarried overlong in foreign

parts, ailments that may end fatally when all hope of return is lost? How often do beautiful maidens and handsome youths, caught in the toils of love, grow ghastly pale and waste away, consumed by melancholy, green-sickness, or erotomania, when delays occur or the hope of possession is lost? These ailments become worse and so much the more difficult for the physician to cure since the underlying affection commonly hides behind the mask of disease and the true source of origin is often difficult to discover. Recent instances might give offense. I take one, therefore, from the older records. Let Perdiccas come forth: inflamed by love of Phila, the concubine of the king his father, he had abandoned all hope of ever possessing her and, having restrained his ardor within, is said to have fallen seriously ill. Nor did he recover until Hippocrates shrewdly observed that as often as Phila came by the pulse beat of the invalid altered, and after having thus uncovered the cause of the disease and prevailed upon the father, rendered him at last partaker of the desire. Plutarch tells a similar story of Antiochus, the son of Seleucus, king of Syria, whose illness, born of love of his father's wife, Stratonice, after it had responded to no remedies whatsoever, Erasistratus, like Hippocrates, at last comprehended and cured with a happy guess and paternal acquiescence to the desire. The fair sex carries the hidden flame of love with no less harm, as is shown by the woman in Galen who languished with desire for the dancer Pylades, and by similar instances today that physicians sometimes uncover to their own advantage.

(26a) Gaub digresses at this point to consider the harmful corporeal effects of unsatisfied desire. The desire is for something thought good, but the harmful emotional reaction is due to its thwarting rather than fulfilment. He first mentions melancholy, green-sickness, and erotomania or love-sickness.[116] Green-sickness and chlorosis were used synonymously in Gaub's time as they are today (although the terms are almost obsolete). A modern medical dictionary describes the condition as one of anemia affecting young girls, associated with digestive and nervous disturbances.[117] Erotomaniacs are defined in an eighteenth-century medical lexicon as those "who engage in the furious pursuit of vagrant and illicit lust".[118] It is nymphomania, in other words, rather than the condition called "insane love" (amor insanus) which is the form apt to hide behind the mask of disease, as Gaub remarks. (26b) The apocryphal story of Hippocrates' shrewd and humane diagnosis of the ailment of Perdiccas is one of the first in a long series. Plutarch's account of Antiochus and Stratonice states that Erasistratus reached his conclusion after observing the flushing, sweating and palpitation of the heart manifested by the unhappy youth in the presence of the object of his desire. By an ingenious stratagem Erasistratus persuaded the king to yield up his wife.[119] Galen, in giving an account of his own somewhat similar case, writes that he is not certain just how Erasistratus made a correct diagnosis. He himself was called to attend a woman suffering from intractable insomnia and melancholy. Refusing to reply to his questions, she turned her face to the wall when he persisted. He thereupon questioned her servant and came to the conclusion she was suffering from a difficulty of mental rather than physical origin, one probably due to grief. After gaining the confidence of the patient to some extent he happened to observe her on her return from a performance by the dancer, Pylades. He noted that her color was good and her pulses full and irregular—the latter the sign, he remarks, of a disturbed mind. Still not satisfied with the evidence he tried the effect of various names on her pulse. She responded only to the name of Pylades and he concluded with certainty that she was suffering from love-sickness. In connection with this and a similar case (a household servant who fell mysteriously ill when asked to give an account of a large sum of money) Galen remarks that other physicians had failed to make the correct diagnoses because they were unaware of the extent to which the body can be affected by emotional disorder.[120] (26c) The literature on the subject of the various forms of illness due to excess of desire is very extensive. We may consider at this point the opinions of some of Gaub's contemporaries. Juncker agrees that love can be a plague to both body and mind, a cause of chlorosis, hysteria and even insanity.[121] Laroque tells us that when young girls fall in love and find themselves unable to satisfy their desires nymphomania may result—indecent gestures and lascivious words leave no doubt in the physician's mind as to their condition, but in most instances he is helpless.[122] Valangin does not mention nymphomania, but he calls thwarted or unsatisfied desire for a loved object one of the most frequent causes of green-sickness in young girls,[123] and Holland, too, refers this condition (which he terms chlorosis) to the same source, remarking that it is a very stubborn ailment.[124] As a physician, writes Zückert, one sees the unfortunate effects on bodily health of unhappy love affairs almost every day. A kind of slow consumption of the body, known to the English as "heartbreak", may result.[125] (26d) Abundant material on the subject of diseases of love may be found in medical writers of the sixteenth and seventeenth centuries, but this need not detain us here. Further comment will be found in the notes.[126]

XII   Harmful Corporeal Effects of Excessive Joy

27. Yet I cannot deny that the cases I have cited here are such as to pertain rather to sorrow or grief resulting from a thwarted appetite for something considered desirable, and that I have not fully proved what I proposed. Let us therefore turn our attention to joy; exulting and revelling in the thought of a present good it is alloyed with no trace of bitterness whatsoever. Would you not suppose, gentlemen,

that this elevated state of the mind is everywhere of benefit to the body and quite without harm? In fact, however, it is sometimes fatal. Not to trouble you with a long list of names I ask you to consult the elder Pliny! Put the question to Gellius! They will tell you of many people who were deprived of life by the sudden onset of unrestrained joy. Guicciardini, the famous Italian historian, relates that Leo, the tenth Pope of that name, was so very pleasurably elated by a greatly desired report of the capture of Milan that he was overcome by a fever and expired a short time thereafter. In our own age it is widely known that the mother of Shah Thamas, king of Persia, disturbed by the civil quarrels of the followers of her son, rejoiced so exceedingly after the report of the defeat and rout of the rebel leader Aszraff by the vigorous commander of the royal army, Thamas Koulikan, that she went out of her mind for several successive days. In truth, man is so fashioned that moderation is the only support and guarantee of the integrity of life and health. No one can bear without harm that which repeatedly and frequently deviates from the uniform course and order of nature. Regardless of whether the mind is moved by the thought of something good or bad, danger of disease or death threatens whenever the excitement disturbs the harmonious course of the bodily economy, as it so often does.

(27a) The bodily effects of love-sickness are caused by a thwarted appetite for something thought good. Gaub now returns to the harmful effects of unrestrained joy, an emotion in which the appetite for something thought good has been satisfied. The story of Pope Leo, which Gaub attributes to Francesco Guicciardini (1483–1540), may also be found in the chapter in Montaigne previously cited as the source of the story of Raisciac.[127] Valangin repeats the story of Leo X in his discussion of the effects of joy[128] and Corp says that excessive happiness injures even healthy people at times, therefore the greatest circumspection is necessary to avoid arousing this emotion in the ill.[129]   Juncker tells a curious story about the nephew and heir of Leibniz who discovered a chest full of coins in the house of his uncle after the latter's death, and was so overcome with delight that he promptly fell dead himself.[130]   Boerhaave gives another such account. A respectable family, reduced to poverty, sent its eldest son to India to recoup the family fortunes.   He soon became wealthy.   Wishing to surprise his sister, he sent for her without further word and on her arrival appeared at the port laden with jewels; she was so overcome with joy that she became suddenly immobile and expired on the spot.[131] (27b) If we turn to Aulus Gellius, as Gaub advises, we find four frequently cited instances of death attributed to excessive and unexpected joy.[132]

XIII   The Corporeal Benefits of Right Reason

28. Forgive me, gentlemen, if, detained by a wealth of material, I have kept you too long in this ghastly battlefield, so to speak, of mankind with its thousands of injuries and fatalities!   And thou, immortal Mind! Forgive me if I have compelled you, man's better part —nay more, his divine part as well, it is said—to sit neglected and accused throughout a long recital of the crimes that you inflict on your companion, the body. I grant indeed that your nature, insofar as it reflects its celestial origin, partakes of all that is pure and untouched by weakness.   But indeed, to mention nothing else, is there not enough to blemish your native purity in the earthly body in which you are held, in the companionship in which you are so artfully joined?   I have already condoled you sufficiently in a special lecture, when I described the ills, disturbances and hindrances inflicted on you by your consort; you were able to deceive yourself, and from this excess of

flattery to believe that all blame for disturbances in the domestic tranquillity fell entirely on the brute body. It is necessary, therefore, to confront you with a mirror in which you may see yourself and your actions, and so learn to recognize the ailments of the body brought about in turn by your persuasion or pressure. It is in fact possible to restore the advantages of conjugal life and the mutual respect of partners only if both of them recognize and admit their guilt. It will be of greater value, I believe, for you yourself to reflect on this matter, and since I seem to sense your repentance I shall take pains to encourage you again and conceal your baseness. Recalling the advantages afforded to bodily health by your energy and foresight, I shall duly honor and embellish your virtue and kindness with statements of praise.

29. I come now, gentlemen, to what I consider essential to the plan of my undertaking: to show that those faculties of the mind which I have so far held to disturb the body frequently and very gravely often help it by providing the most powerful safeguards— a subject that I so much the more willingly undertake to the extent that it provides more pleasant and advantageous things to be uttered and heard, one that also allows my discourse to rejoice and triumph in the cause of the mind. The services that I am to celebrate here are indeed so numerous and important that I do not shrink from the claim that no power in the whole of nature more effectively preserves the health of the body or restores it when it fails. What I say may perhaps sound exaggerated and unbelievable to you. But, indeed, if anyone more carefully reflects on my demonstration of how greatly the mind can variously alter the state of the body, so that absolutely none of the motive powers, functions, interior organs and humors can resist its force, he will, unless I am much mistaken, find it very difficult to believe that a power of the mind so great is always disastrous in its effects

and harmful under all circumstances, rather than to consider, by a legitimate inference that it is equally capable of bringing about the good and operating to the advantage of the bodily economy, in accord with circumstances. Ask physicians who teach from wide experience that the harshest measures may in practice often be the most wholesome, that one disease may prevent, moderate or cure another, that there are remedies which finally bring about a happy cure only after having excited diseases, that there are many others which safely relieve the ill but greatly harm the sound and healthy, that there are still others which hardly affect the well yet harm the ill, and, lastly, that the most dangerous poisons may overcome diseases resistant to all other remedies when administered with care and caution while, on the other hand, the best remedies are converted into deadly poisons when inopportunely used. Since these things are quite true and fully support my position, I could rest content with this kind of showing did not the importance of the subject and the scope of my discourse demand a more complete demonstration.

30. The first instance from which one can see that a tranquil mind making use of right reason aids the health in many ways is that it adjusts and regulates both its own functions and those attributable to the body in such a way that the organs are neither sluggish as a result of inactivity nor worn out by too much work, the natural needs being properly attended to and anything known to be in any way detrimental carefully avoided. Is there anyone who wants proof in words when his own experience and the example of countless others impressively teach that nothing is more unhealthy than an immoderate way of life? I ask you, gentlemen, to recall once again the ailments which I have just mentioned, as numerous as they are dangerous, arising solely from the emotions! Look about you! The eye is everywhere struck by the fate of gluttons,

drunkards, lechers and others of the company of intemperates! How often they die before their time, their powers exhausted by debauchery, or are not only already senile when barely middle-aged but go from one illness to another and drag out a life to which death would be preferable! The old age which Cicero praises in the elder Cato was far different. That, I say, was the close of a life in accord with the precepts of reason, a close approaching so slowly and gently, in consequence of the temperance carefully practiced throughout the preceding stages of life, that the greybeard feels himself to have lived for a long time rather than to have become aged. Hence one may observe that many men of average circumstances enjoy the better fate, being neither marred at birth by the vices of their parents nor weakened by a soft upbringing: obtaining sufficient food and clothing to satisfy their natural needs by means of fitting employment, passing peacefully through life free from care and content with their own affairs, incited neither to overindulgence by riches nor by ambition to violent emotions, their sound health rarely disturbed by disease, they bring their long lives to a close, finished not so much by the weariness of old age as by its inflexibility. Do you wish me, gentlemen, to mention in addition how much a serene state of mind does for the ill? How injurious are impatience, fretfulness and lack of self-restraint? The harm to themselves and the numerous therapeutic difficulties for physicians occasioned by those who resist all measures and correctly observe nothing prescribed to be followed or shunned? Shall I recount the numerous advantages that the sick and infirm, recovering from an illness, are wont to praise when each one, on the basis of his own experience, establishes a way of life in accord with nature to which he scrupulously adheres, the mind attentive to whatever is helpful or harmful? This would be superfluous in a matter so well known to all, and I would act to no purpose were I now to refute at length those who are compelled by desire, rather than taught by reason, to think otherwise. Let them recall the proverb; *To live medically is to live miserably*, and console themselves with it when at last, too late, they come to their senses. If you will permit me, I shall cite only one witness for the case, one beyond all exception. A Venetian nobleman, Luigi Cornaro, who was given to extravagant debauchery as a young man, in keeping with his wealth and the customs of the times, so greatly weakened his natural powers that from his twenty-fifth to his fortieth year he struggled on to no purpose, almost continually ill, after having tried in vain every kind of remedy. At last, following the advice of his physicians, he derived so much benefit from the adoption of a very strict mode of life that not only did he find himself free from chronic illness within a year's time but—continuing from then on in the same abstemious course—prolonged a flourishing life to the ultimate human limits, supported by a sound mind and body rather than worn out or enfeebled by senility, and when more than one hundred years of age he died the easy and placid death (*euthanasia*) longed for. Let the differences in outcome show whether it is better to follow the bait of pleasure or the prudent advice of the physician.

(28) That the human mind is part of the divine mind was a tenet of Stoic philosophy. Gaub may have read the statement in Cicero.[133] In the first lecture he rejected the belief that the mind was a prisoner in the body, and we may perhaps regard the Platonic and Plotinic overtones of his remarks here as rhetorical in intent. (29) Having mildly admonished the "mind" for failing to recognize her shortcomings Gaub will now show how greatly she benefits the body. The power to destroy is also the power to preserve, and in order to support his claim that the same agency may have both beneficial and harmful effects on the body

he draws several analogies based on the cure of one disease by another, the remedial action of poisons, and the poisonous action of remedies, topics which were presumably familiar to his auditors.[134] (30a) The "first service" rendered by mind to body comes from the tranquil mind acting in accord with the dictates of right reason, and the service itself is the optimum regulation of mental and physical functions. The examples given later on—drunkards, lechers and others of the company of intemperates[135]—and the phrase "right reason" give the clue to sources of Gaub's thought which are again to be found in Cicero. The *Tusculan Disputations* contain a lengthy treatment of intemperance (using the Latin term *intemperantia* just as Gaub does). Cicero calls intemperance a revolt against right reason, followed by a release of the appetites.[136] In reading Cicero and Gaub we must be careful to distinguish between the two meanings of intemperance: on the one hand an imbalance of the fluid but corporeal components of the body, i.e. dyscrasia, on the other imbalance of the mind. Gaub, like most medical writers, desires to point out the interdependence of the two. Cicero tells us in the *Tusculan Disputations* that the Stoics compare the disorder of the mind characteristic of the one kind of intemperance with corporeal disorders characterized by humoral imbalance,[137] in other words they compare disease of the mind with disease of the body. Furthermore, just as men by virtue of their individual corporeal temperaments are prone to certain bodily diseases, so are they, by virtue of their mental temperament, prone to certain emotional disorders.[138] We have previously noted that Cicero translated the Greek term *sôphrosynê* by the Latin *temperantia*,[139] Galen, in discussing the emotions, uses the term *sôphrosynê* in the same way,[140] and in the pseudo-Galenical *Medical Definitions* health, strength, beauty and wholeness of the body are compared with prudence, temperance (*sôphrosynê*), fortitude and justice of the mind.[141] Similarly, Cicero finds that beauty, health, strength and vigor of the body are matched by corresponding features of the mind; *temperatio* of the body is analogous to *temperatio*

of the mind.[142]   Concern with *sôphrosynê* makes its first
and perhaps greatest appearance in the Platonic dialogue
Charmides.[143]   Applying to Socrates for a cure of his
headache Charmides is told that the Greek physicians know
that the head cannot be treated apart from the whole body,
but they do not know that the body (*sôma*) cannot be treated
apart from the mind (*psychê*)—and this he had learned, said
Socrates, from a Thracian while on a military campaign.
The Thracian had told him further that everything good or
bad in the body originated in the mind, and that the proper
treatment of the mind required the use of words to engender
temperance (*sôphrosynê*).   The great error of our day in the
treatment of human beings, said the Thracian, is that men
try to treat health and temperance separately.[144]   (30b)
The term euthanasia, applied here in the case of Cornaro,
means an easy natural death rather than one induced by the
physician or the State in cases of incurable painful disease
or mental defect.   From the theological standpoint it means
the happy and placid death of one whose faith is assured.[145]
Luigi Cornaro (1467-1566) is said to have restricted himself at first to a diet of twelve ounces of solid food and fourteen ounces of wine; later he found that an egg sufficed for a
day's solid food.   He wrote four treatises on the subject
of attaining a long life at the ages of eighty-three, eighty-six,
ninety-one and ninety-five, respectively, the first of which
went through several editions in English.   He died in
Padua at the age of ninety-eight.[146]   (30c) Pechlin offers
his opinion as a physician that the fearless and prudent can
expect euthanasia; he has only contempt for those who
"flee to the shadow with unbecoming groans".[147]

XIV Quasi-Rational, Instinctive, Benefits to the Body; The Problem of the Healing Powers of Nature

31. So much for the first kind of service that the mind performs for the body. I come now to the second, and I must confess that I do not know how to designate it properly. In both the well and the ill it is evident on certain occasions that definite movements, urges and appetites, different from the usual course and order of nature, manifest themselves. Since they originate in parts of the body where the mind exercises control we would seem well advised to hold that they should be referred back to the mind itself as the source from which they flow. Seeing that they appear to be deliberately carried out with an underlying aim toward the health of the body, to the pursuit of which many are quite appropriate, one might indeed hold that they arise with the help of reason and, further, that they are worked out with unique foresight, the aid given having been called for by the mind in order to preserve life's integrity. If we consider on the other hand that the mind is at such times unaware of any plan or purpose, and that these events occur not only in the discerning but to an equal degree in the most uncultivated, to whom the power of rational thought is denied by age, natural deficit or mode of life, a legitimate doubt arises whether this efficacy is indeed rightly to be attributed to the mind. It so happens that something similar shows itself even more clearly in living creatures that, according to prevailing opinion, lack the use of reason. Since philosophers can neither derive these happenings from the body nor ascribe them to a plan or purpose, they take refuge in some, I know not what, instinct, which signifies something quasi-rational and analogous to reason, or at all events expresses in one term every effect that seems to

be derived from the same unknown principle. But these matters are foreign to the medical forum, and I touch on them only lightly so that you will understand the kind of movement I intend to discuss in more detail insofar as it occurs in man, and will thus be able to ascribe it properly to the mind.

32. My talk would never end were I to set forth here each and every point of importance and enumerate and exalt the benefits derived by the body from this source, in accordance with their merits. There are indeed so many that it is difficult to imagine greater, and were they lacking there would be neither stability with regard to the many necessities of life nor protection against the many agents injurious to the health. I shall, therefore, mention only a few from a great number. To begin at birth, what is more important to the life of the newborn infant when it first comes to the light and thereafter to man at every stage of growth, than breathing? Do you hold that the body of its own accord initiates breathing? Even though an answer to this question is still lacking, it is more likely the mind. Almost all physiologists agree that an awareness of some difficulty or need compels the newborn in this direction, and that respiration is among those functions which the mind governs and regulates in accordance with judgement. It is accompanied by crying and screaming, and an infant perhaps exhausted by the act of delivery who is remiss in starting may be caused to breathe by external stimulation. Who does not know that second only to his need for air man can least afford to do without food? Immediately after birth the untutored infant brought to the maternal breast at once begins without difficulty to suck and swallow the milk prepared for it. This act is accomplished by muscles under voluntary control, and it is therefore the mind that of its own free will—or, if you prefer, autodidact and under the influence of some instinct or other—meets the needs of the body by this

maneuver. If it had first to be learned, like walking and talking, which of us would have survived to leave the cradle?

33. Shortness of time forces me to omit many other such matters. Frequently overlooked because they occur every day and are common to the universe of living beings, they are nevertheless of such outstanding utility that in their absence human life—I say the entire race of man—would soon come to an end. Those seen in the ill are most worthy of mention. As true friendship is given its final test in adversity, so the mind gives the most impressive evidence of its love for the body only when nature is burdened by disease and driven to the wall. Hence you see that even the prodigal sons, whose vicious mode of life while still healthy would, you will say, suggest that they have at heart nothing more than a concern for the ruin of their bodies, search anxiously for aid and leave nothing untried that may restore them to grace and health once they attain their desire and fall ill. Doubtless the disagreeable experience of pain, anguish or debility so stirs up the mind that it is driven to seek for a remedy even against its will, and not uncommonly those who hold the art of medicine in mockery or contempt fly to the physician at the onset of illness, humbly prepared to plead error in excuse. It is just this restless concern of the mind with an afflicted body that leads the ill to prefer to try something doubtful or dangerous rather than to do nothing at all when a safe remedy, recommended by reason and science, is wanting. It is this that impels those who are troubled by incurable ailments to try the uncertain, even against medical advice, and to use one remedy after another without caution, with the result that they fall into a worse state, either increasing their miseries or hastening their death. In this same way the most untutored peoples once learned of herbs and other modalities helpful in the treatment of wounds and disease, so that though

without physicians they were by no means without remedies, and this seems to be the original source of the medical art.

34. Perhaps you may hold that what I have presented suggests the advice and direction of reason rather than instinct. The matter cannot be argued here as it might, since I have that which is plainer and quite without ambiguity. I shall not touch on the fact that respiration undergoes a multitude of changes in accordance with different bodily states and that disturbances of the bodily economy are alleviated by increased or decreased movement, by coughing, sneezing, yawning, sighing, and in many other ways—yet just consider a man who is troubled by a respiratory difficulty and marvel at the way in which the mind not only carefully adjusts the position of the body and the arrangement of its members but also directs all strength of the voluntary muscles so as to afford help when life is in danger! Again, let a man contract a fever from some inner corruption. If the sufferer, weak after several days of fasting, is offered foods of animal origin—meat, fish, eggs, or soups prepared from them—he will abruptly reject everything. He will be nauseated, disgusted and distressed by the odor alone. Such foods are indeed by nature prone to spontaneous decay and so quickly corrupted when they reach a stomach already tainted by decay that they add fire to the evil rather than give nourishment. A prudent aversion, of great help to the ailing, one worthy of being claimed for its own by sound reason! Yet the wise and the most stupid, the dull and the knowing, the child and the adult have it in common; moreover it manifests itself even in the insane and in brute beasts. What more shall I say? The mind is not content with avoiding the harmful, for the same instinct also leads it to conceive very healthy appetites which make the source of origin clear to the physician, pointing with a finger, as it were, toward the kinds of remedies needed. A man parched

by internal heat or insatiable thirst longs for fluids, for cool, sour, restorative drinks, above all else, and when allowed to drink them at his pleasure he does so avidly and is marvellously refreshed, as if he had been taught that nothing else could more surely quench the fire, soothe the sharpness, and prevent putridity. The services of the mind extend even further. The insatiable desire for acids present while the disease flourishes grows weaker when it declines and changes into aversion when it is fully overcome, whereas the appetite for what had been distasteful returns. Otherwise the prostrate powers could not recover nor could a defect in the humors contrary to the first one be avoided. If I were to wish now to add to this the extraordinary urges toward the consumption of the unusual and even highly disagreeable displayed at times by pregnant women, the aversions to foods and drinks with which a harmful excess of humors is safely and gently warded off, if I were to bring forth the palid virgins who suffer from acidity and delight excessively in absorbent earths, if I were to cite the instances of men who, after fighting a long and tedious battle with illness relieved neither by nature nor the art of medicine, are happily saved at last by the immoderate consumption of something vehemently desired as the result of an appetite arising spontaneously, your patience would be more quickly exhausted than my material.

(31) In the previous paragraph Gaub dealt with matters which clearly lay within the domain of mind, since they involved the rational choice by the person concerned of modes of life most conducive to health. Now the course of his argument becomes rather uncertain, as he proceeds to ascribe more to "mind" than his original principles allowed. We recall that in his first lecture he defined mind as the realm of thought[148] and that he frequently spoke so as to imply that it was coextensive with awareness. Now he

places certain activities, impulses and desires of seemingly purposeful character—although there is no awareness of purpose associated with the actions as carried out—in the realm of mind on the ground that they originate in parts of the body where conscious control is or can be exerted. They have nothing to do with rationality as generally understood, yet they take place in such a way as to suggest the operation of "unique foresight", hence philosophers have ascribed them to instinct.[149] (32) Respiration is the first of the relevant bodily activities to be mentioned. Gaub believes respiration cannot be called a purely corporeal function because the voluntary musculature is involved and many physiologists of his day claim that some degree of awareness and exercise of judgement is required (eighteenth-century physiologists were apt to concern themselves with problems that would today be assigned to the psychologist). The second activity has to do with the taking of food early in life. The infant makes use, without prior instruction, of muscles considered to be under voluntary control when it takes the breast and sucks. It seems to be Gaub's opinion that to call these movements instinctive classifies them neatly but hides the problem behind a word, judging from his offhand references to "instinct" in this and the preceding paragraph. (33) Gaub calls attention here to a kind of half blind, instinctive striving toward health manifested by the human being in the face of illness. It leads the sick man to turn in every direction for help and to try one remedy after another. This urge may have deleterious effects, but on the other hand it may lead to the discovery of the appropriate remedy. The art of medicine is itself, he says, the result of some such striving. (34a) The first sentence is rather puzzling, since Gaub has already called instinct "quasi-rational". Furthermore, he did not state that he intended to exclude examples that suggested the operation of instinct (nor does he). (34b) Clinical observation had no doubt taught Gaub how quickly a patient learns to adjust his positions or motions in accordance with the requirements of his disease, e.g. the patient with heart disease learns to sleep in a sitting position and thereby avoid dangerous respiratory disturbance, and the patient with pleurisy to avoid pain by splinting the affected side. The choice of reason is clearly evident here, but not so in the next group of examples. It may indeed happen that a sufferer rejects some item of diet because he knows of its effects from experience, yet the aversion to a particular food often stems from a deeper and not readily explicable source, as we see from its occurrence in the insane and in "brute beasts". The healthy appetites conceived by the mind are often nicely adjusted to avoid both excesses and defects in the body fluids. Gaub allows physiological significance to the abnormal appetites conceived by pregnant women,[150] to the consumption of absorbent earths by "pallid virgins" (presumably to neutralize an excess of acid), and to the spontaneous curative appetites sometimes observed in the ill. (34c) In order to understand the full significance of Gaub's remarks we must undertake an extended presentation of his conception of the healing power of nature, chiefly as set forth in the chapter of the *Institutiones* devoted to that topic, but drawing from the entire book. Life, health, disease, and death, Gaub tells us, are the four natural events that chiefly concern the physician. Although the first two are conditions according to nature[151] and the last conditions against nature, or praeternatural conditions,[152] all come under the wider meaning of the word "nature". To call an event "natural", Gaub writes, is simply to say that it has physical causes which determine its origin, duration, activities and decline, causes coming from without or seated within.[153] In the human body life and health are furthered and disease and death hindered by the action of the human mind, which operates both consciously and by means of "blind instinct".[154] Man finds himself situated in the world in relation to innumerable things, each with its proper power of action and all in perpetual flux and change; he cannot always forego, avoid, or adjust these things to his liking. Whether arising from within or coming from without they affect the body and thereby the mind.

Favorably or unfavorably they arouse, suppress or otherwise act on the natural powers and are acted upon in turn.[155] Are we justified, Gaub asks, in retaining the ancient idea of disease as a "contest of nature"[156] in which Nature asserts her powers and preserves the health? This belief has been held and approved by the wisest masters of the art of medicine, he tells us, and there is in fact a never-sleeping power of human nature[157] perpetually engaged in securing the necessary and warding off the harmful. This power is the source of the spontaneous, unwilled, bodily movements that constitute the so-called *molimina* of disease. The *molimina* are events in the body that must be distinguished from disease, from the causes of disease, and from the effects of the physician's remedies. Many of them are so aptly directed toward the restoral of health that nothing more appropriate could be devised by art. It is, then, rightly taught that nature is the physician of diseases and the physician the servant of nature.[158] The sum of the art of medicine is the observation, imitation and direction of nature. These golden words ought always to be kept before the eyes of physicians. Yet it is wrong to swallow them down too hastily, for those who suppose that nothing but good comes from this source are mistaken. Nature makes mistakes. Her impetuous actions may be misdirected, harmful or even fatal. The prudent physician is to do more than act as a marvelling and approving spectator. He must restrain the efforts of Nature when she is over-precipitate, arouse her when she is too torpid and bring her back to the right path when she goes astray. Nature's victory is rarely without wounds.[159]

The idea of a contest, Gaub says, implies an adversary, and this adversary is the disease itself. If you mistake the therapeutic efforts of Nature for the disease will you say that disease is absent when Nature gives up the struggle? Will you call the changes brought about by the physician's remedies disease? It is true that the natural therapeutic endeavors often constitute a major part of the symptoms and signs of disease. Sometimes diseases change their character when the *molimina* supervene, and the latter must be carefully distinguished from the disease proper. As for the terminological question, Gaub suggests that we follow Hippocrates and speak simply of the natural healing powers. To attempt to replace this phrase with *anima*, *archeus*, or the designation of any other rational or quasi-rational principle leads to a dispute about words rather than facts.[160] The new words shed no further light on the subject and there is no reason to prefer them to the old.[161] Gaub attempts to distinguish the protective activities of the mind from such activities occurring automatically in consequence of the arrangement of the bodily parts. Man has a mind which is capable of directing its powers in the body against the enemy, disease. When damage is inflicted on the body the mind is aroused and made anxious and these powers are activated. The body, too, is so constituted that when one part is injured the others often combine their powers and hasten to its aid. Since nature is often unable to keep such defensive activities within the limits defining the state of health, they may at times give rise to disturbances greater than those excited by the disease itself. The "defensive efforts" (*molimina*) include derangements of the appetite, aversions for certain foods, spasmodic movements, convulsions, abnormal movements of the humors, fever, eruptions of the skin, abscess formation, hemorrhage, vomiting, diarrhea, sweating and many more.[162] Man, Gaub continues, comes in contact with so large a number of noxious agents that it is almost impossible for him to remain free from disease throughout his life. The human body, exposed as it is to the ceaseless activities of daily life, would soon be worn away and destroyed by the movements of its parts had it not the power to appropriate materials to itself from the outside world. With these materials it preserves itself intact in the face of the perpetual flux and change of its corporeal substance. It has, likewise, various powers effective against the unavoidable causes of disease and death. Included among the bodily powers is a wonderful ability to restore wounds, fractures, ulcers, injuries and mutilations. Nature displays marvellous skill here, and the whole art of surgery rests on the basis of her efforts.[163]   It was standard humoral doctrine in Gaub's time that disease-producing, corrupt or harmful matter (called *materia peccans*) in the body was subjected to "coctions", and thus readied for external disposal or convenient disposition within.   By expulsion of the harmful matter, or by its removal to a more convenient place in or on the body, the original healthy balance of the humors was restored.[164]   To this process of coction Gaub applied the alternative Greek term *pepasmos*.[165]   He drew an implicit analogy between the power of the body to digest and assimilate food and its power to "subdue and commingle" harmful or praeternatural agencies acting against the body.   The beneficial effects observed in the crises of disease depended on this ability of the body to mitigate, make innocuous, or expel harmful things tending toward or causing disease.[166]   Suppuration, i.e. the formation of pus, was one of the most outstanding of the manifestations of *pepasmos*.   In the absence of this process wounds, ulcers and inflammations could not be healed.[167]   Gaub pointed out that in disposing of harmful agencies or substances the normal expulsive passages of the body were sometimes used, but more often than not unusual ways and means were called into action.   There are many motive powers of the body that can be aroused by noxious agencies in such a way as to protect life and health.   Among them are certain automatic and self-maintaining bodily movements (using the term movement in its broadest sense) which, although often irregular, are usually beneficial and tend to produce a healthy outcome.   They cannot be attributed to the mind because they often occur in the absence of awareness, or against the will.   Among these "movements" Gaub includes fever. He admits that fever is a severe disturbance of the bodily economy, associated with a derangement of the circulatory system, and that it may be harmful or even disastrous in some instances.   Yet it is at times so beneficial that no more certain and powerful aid is to be found in art or

nature.[168]   Physicians, he says, have joined their voices in
praising fever and have often regretted that they could not
induce it as easily as expel it.[169]

In addition to the various protective activities or "movements" carried out solely by the body, the human mind,
Gaub reminds us again, strives to preserve bodily health.[170]
The disagreeable awareness of a threatening ill or the
recollection of one once suffered often impel us to seek for
remedies and safeguards.   Reason, experience and con-
jecture are called on for aid.   At a lower level, the mind
incites movements in the body.   Some of these, Gaub
admits, seem to have an instinctive or quasi-rational rather
than a rational source, yet their scope and efficacy is nonetheless remarkable.   Certain spontaneous movements of the
muscles ordinarily under control of the will fall into this
class as do spontaneous distastes and appetites.   By yielding
to these movements, appetites and aversions a threatening
disease may sometimes be averted or a refractory disease
cured.   Finally, Gaub calls our attention to the remarkable
power of adapting to circumstances possessed by both mind
and body.   We become hardened by custom to innumerable harmful things.   Custom renders even diseases more
tolerable and tractable; it mitigates the effects of poisons
themselves.   Hence the time-worn observation that old
bad habits are often less harmful than good new ones.
This is the sum and substance of the natural healing powers,
Gaub concludes.   By virtue of these powers health is more
common, on the whole, than disease, and many men are
rarely afflicted, while others enjoy uninterrupted health
into old age and a great number recover from illness without
any medical treatment whatsoever, solely as a result of the
operation of these powers.   The art of medicine depends on
the healing powers of nature.   In the absence of these powers
the physician could neither preserve health nor cure disease.
Therefore the physician who learns to make proper use of
the healing powers of nature attains the peak of the art of
medicine.[171]   Where some writers[172] argue that the
question at issue is whether these activities derive from the

operations of the bodily machine in accordance with mechanical laws or are the effects of an extraneous agency called "nature"—passing over the problem of the intervention of mind in bodily events—Gaub takes it for granted that physical causes determine "natural" processes in the human body. He has another problem. The facts themselves are not disputed, he writes, since they are matters of observation open to everyone, but there is endless disagreement about their source. Do they derive exclusively from man's corporeal part or from his mental part? Both views have as proponents outstanding men who dispute vigorously yet are unable to conquer and cannot themselves be overcome. It is plain, Gaub says, that nothing stronger than probable grounds of belief can be offered by either side, hence there is little hope that this dispute can be ended. We labor under a threefold ignorance of the structure and powers of the body, of the nature of the mind and its faculties, and of the fundamental laws of mutual intercourse between the two. Gaub's own opinion is that both mind and body have their peculiar powers of action. Certainly, he claims, there are motive powers in the body independent of those in the mind. In addition to the many activities taking place without awareness or against the will we can observe movements in surviving portions of living bodies. In the former respect the intelligent and the foolish, the infant and the adult, do not differ greatly and indeed this kind of instinctive movement occurs in animals and plants. The rational aspect of the mind does not control the production of *molimina* any more than it does the course of emotional disturbances. Appetites and aversions often seem to be forced on the mind by the ailing body in accordance with the laws determining the definite changes aroused by definite thoughts. Gaub's last word on the subject is that everyone should embrace the opinion he finds most appropriate or, better yet, allow the question to rest undecided. Pathologists and practitioners need concern themselves no further with it until a clear explanation is furnished by the physiologists.[173]

XV   Violent Emotions Compared with Atmospheric Storms

35. This topic has detained me long enough, and it remains only to be shown that the emotions, however much they deviate from right reason, are frequently of great benefit to the body by the very power with which they prevail.   As physicists point out, storms and hurricanes, which rage through the skies with thunder and lightning, lead to a remarkable cleansing of the air, although often destructive.   So these storms, as it were, of the human economy are likewise not so invariably harmful that they do not occasionally have a most beneficial effect on the health as well.

(35) The comparison of physiological disturbances with those of the weather, of emotional storms with atmospheric storms, is no more than metaphorical in Gaub, but we can look back on a time when it was more nearly literal, i.e. when physiological disturbances and meteorological disturbances were both regarded as disturbances in balance of the elementary qualities, hot, cold, moist and dry.   A discussion of this topic will be found in the notes.[174]

XVI   Beneficial Corporeal Effects of Hope in Connection with Various Ailments

36. The less violent emotions which are generated by the thought of some present or future good do indeed benefit the healthy as much as they relieve the ill, and this is so well known and obvious that someone who undertook to doubt it or to demonstrate it in detail would merit no hearing.   The most salutary of all, hope, not only arouses the mind but breathes strength into all of the bodily powers as well.   Hence the misery of old age which, when it forbids distant

hopes to arise, is not sustained even by immediate ones. Hence the sufferers from homesickness who are revivified by hope alone when first they ready themselves to return to their native lands.   Recall, gentlemen, the story told of Democritus, the philosopher of Abdera.   Enfeebled by age, his powers now failing, his grieving sister forced to be absent for three days at the festival of the Goddess Ceres, he is said to have been kept alive by the odor of warm bread long enough until the rites were finished and she could return to care for the dying man, whereupon he then quite peacefully expired.   But, since instances of death delayed by hope are reported in our own day, which of you, I ask, will doubt that the prolongation of the life of the philosopher ought to be attributed not to bread placed before the nose but to hope and desire for a sister about to return? It is this faith that physicians so greatly wish for, since if they know how to procure it for themselves from the ill they render them more obedient and are able to breathe new life into them with words alone, moreover they find the power of their remedies to be increased and the results made more certain.   From this same source quacks, travelling venders of medicine, uroscopists and urine-boilers, who play tricks with charms, amulets and sympathetic powers, seek fame and fortune.   For when they display their prodigies and confidently promise recovery to the ill, with high-flown words and rash boasts, credulity is seized by wonder and wonder leads to hope, which then buoys up a mind enfeebled by an obstinate tedious ailment and want of help.   The arousal of the bodily organs is sometimes such that the vital principles cast off their torpidity, the tone of the nervous system is restored, the movements of the humors are accelerated, and nature then attacks and overcomes with her own powers a disease that prolonged treatment has opposed in vain.   Let those fortunate enough to have more rapidly recovered by means of these empty arts than by means of approved systems of healing congratulate themselves, I say, on having regained their health, regardless of the reason! But if they contend in earnest that this service is to be attributed to the special effects of such remedies they will indeed move experts to laughter and merit no reply.

(36a) In keeping with the scheme given in the first lecture we may regard the action of hope as follows: the *enormôn* of the mind is roused by the belief or judgement which forms the basis of the emotion (in this case hope), the arousal is then communicated to that part of the *enormôn* of the body (the voluntary nervous system) governing voluntary movement and sensation, whereupon the *enormôn* controlling the natural and vital functions (the sympathetic nervous system) is then affected; the end result is that the revivified "natural powers" attack and overcome a disease that had long resisted medical treatment. The statement that the tone of the nervous system is restored[175] refers to a restoral of the forces of contraction and relaxation governed by the nervous system.[176] (36b) Gaub uses the term *nostalgia* for homesickness.[177] It can be cured, he says, by hope alone. We may conveniently discuss this condition here. It was taken much more seriously by physicians then than it is today. One of the frequent causes of protracted severe grief is homesickness, Corp writes, and in Switzerland especially the attachment of young men to their native soil is so great that when forced to leave for service in the army they are sometimes subject to a state of extreme dejection in which they lose health and strength and even die. He gives in detail a report by Dr. Hamilton of Ipswich. The patient, a recruit in the British army, was placed on the sick list because of complaints of weakness, giddiness, noise in the ears, bad dreams, insomnia and melancholy. In spite of medical treatment he continued to waste away in the hospital. Dr. Hamilton at first thought that the patient might be suffering from incipient typhus fever but no further signs of it developed and the usual measures brought no improvement. After three months the recruit is said to have looked like a man in the last stages of consumption: his eyes were hollow, his cheeks prominent; he had frequent night sweats and he was too weak to get in or out of bed without help. One morning the nurse happened to mention to Hamilton the patient's constant talk of home and his friends—which she regarded as the "common ravings of sickness and delirium". Hamilton immediately promised the patient that he could return home (in Wales) on furlough as soon as he was better. Thereafter the promised furlough was discussed on every occasion of the doctor's visit and the patient was at the same time encouraged to eat. His appetite soon mended and after two months he was able to return to the barracks. Hamilton informed the officers of the method of cure and warned them that a relapse was sure to occur if the promised furlough was not obtained. A request was then made to the commanding officer; he "obligingly granted" the furlough.[178] The causes, symptoms and neurophysiology of homesickness were the subject of a dissertation by Johann Harder, the originator of the term "nostalgia". This condition, he wrote, also known as *Heimweh* or *maladie du pays*, had no proper medical name. Since no one had heretofore studied it as carefully as he, he felt that it was also incumbent on him to devise a new name; he proposed "nostalgia", from the Greek *nostos*, a return home (the paper reads *nosos*, disease, but this is clearly a typographical error), and *algos*, pain or sorrow. Others were at liberty to prefer the terms *nosimanias*, or *philopatridomanias*. Nostalgia, continues Harder, is a symptom of a lesion of the imagination due to the constant movement of the animal spirits through the white tubules of the tracts of the striate bodies and the oval center of the brain. The repeated movement of these corporeal spirits along the same paths in the brain excites in the mind a recurring idea of a return home.[179] Some say that the disease is endemic in Switzerland, especially in Berne, but this is not true. Harder states that there are various remote, internal and predisposing causes which arouse in the mind the idea of returning home. The external antecedent causes are differences in climate, customs, habits and food, insults and injuries, and many others. It is not difficult to understand how the symptoms arise, he claims. The fixed idea (in the mind) of returning home fixes (in the brain) the course of the animal spirits, which then become sluggish in their movements and cannot sustain the "vibration of fibrils in the common sensorium" necessary for other acts of the mind. For the same reason the spirits also, being too busied in the brain, do not flow in sufficient quantity and force through the tubules of the nerves to the other parts of the body, and therefore cannot assist their natural activities. The appetite is dulled, the gastric flow becomes sluggish, food is imperfectly digested, and a "cruder chyle" mixes with the blood to produce a viscid serum poor in animal spirits. Since the animal spirits are regenerated in insufficient quantity on the one hand, and consumed in excess in the brain on the other, the natural and voluntary motions grow torpid, languor spreads throughout the body and the circulation of the blood grows weak. The blood becomes thicker and more apt to coagulate, the heart moves more sluggishly and the blood-vessels distend. This leads to anxiety, low grade fever and obstruction of glands by viscid, crude and acid serum. The consumption of the spirits and ensuing weakness of the body hasten death.[180] Zückert, writing seventy-odd years later, says that homesickness (*Heimweh*, *Heimsehnsucht*, *nostalgia* and *pathopatridalgia*) is a disease whose cause will be sought for in vain in altered conditions of climate and air, since it is clearly the result of an emotional disturbance. Accompanying the mental depression typical of the disease are bodily symptoms such as tremors and wasting, and even death may result.[181] (36c) As for the beneficial effects of hope itself, Corp devotes an entire chapter to the subject. It energizes the nervous system, invigorates the heart and circulation, and maintains the tension of the blood-vessels. He points out that hope has prophylactic value in connection with epidemic diseases. During outbreaks of plague we should, he says, fortify the minds of those who are exposed to the disease by convincing them that the disease is not incurable and seeing that they do not become too depressed by the death of others. Physicians are not to be censured for trying to cultivate hope in their patients to the last. They may otherwise both hasten the exit of the sick and render their last moments more miserable. The physician can be quite mistaken in his prognosis, and persons may recover on the brink of the grave who probably would not have escaped death had they been given the physician's opinion of their danger.[182] Corp also quotes Boerhaave and van Swieten to the effect that hope may help cure certain fevers by accelerating the movement of the humors.[183] (36d) Diogenes Laertius gives a less sentimental version of the story. The sister of Democritus was vexed by the possibility that he would die during the festival and that a premature return would prevent her from offering fitting worship, but by applying hot loaves to his nostrils Democritus managed to outlive the celebration.[184] (36e) As for the cures performed by quacks, Corp says that in the "rude times of medical science" amulets, incantations and charms were much in use, and he can well imagine that salutary changes in the bodily economy were thus produced. If, he adds, in the present enlightened age we find persons who believe in the efficacy of charms or modes of cure equally ridiculous, it will, "I think, be proper to make use of such remedies . . . at the same time, however, it will be highly necessary to administer such medicines as are most likely to effect a cure, taking care that the patient considers them merely as auxiliaries, otherwise real remedies may be wholly rejected." He notes some diseases, such as consumption, in which the hopes of the patient remain delusively high to the end.[185] Everyday observation, Pechlin tells us, shows that the degree of faith aroused by the physician determines the effectiveness of his treatment.[186] The power of the imagination to produce disease is also plain enough. This comes about by the transformation of an incorporeal idea into its corporeal exemplar. The strongly held idea is communicated to the animal spirits, thence to the vital spirits, and thence to the humors and solid part of the body.   In this way a disease of the mind is transformed to one of the body.[187]   Pechlin finds the power of the mind to influence bodily processes of the kind taking place in diseases not much more remarkable than the power exerted over the voluntary muscles by mimes, actors and acrobats.[188]   The older writers have much to say on this subject, and their opinions are rarely as naïve as generally believed.[189]

XVII   Beneficial Corporeal Effects of Joy, Faith and Love

37. No less curative power is present in joy.   What is told of Peiresc, a noble-minded French Maecenas of former times, by his biographer Gassendi is first of all worth recalling.   He was stricken by a severe paralysis that spread from his leg to involve the entire right side of his body including the tongue itself, so that he lost all power of articulate speech.   He is said, on first receiving a letter from his dearest friend, de Thou, and then on hearing a certain hymn sung in a most delightful fashion, to have experienced such rapture that while exulting and striving to utter the words— Oh how beautiful it is!—he did in fact utter them, whereupon he immediately recovered free use of all members.

38. I have pointed out above that love can derange the health, with instances which show likewise that it can even replace medicine if the desired object is attained.   Nature itself once taught the ancient peoples of the East that feeble and worn out old men are marvellously restored when warmed by lying with a young girl.   But anyone who believes that the whole effect lies only in the enticing warmth that flows from the young body and attributes nothing to the spark of love, however fleeting, struck at the same time will find it difficult to explain why the warmth of the fair sex is

preferred. How much more happy would the physician be in curing diseases of virgins if whenever need arose he took opportune advantage of the counsel of Hippocrates—let the virgin unite with a man!

(37a) The reference here is to Pierre Gassendi's life of N. F. de Peiresc.[190]   The story of de Peiresc may also be found in Pechlin, together with another instance of the beneficial effects of joy.   Women half dead with pain after a difficult delivery forget everything when given their infants.[191]   (37b) Valangin relays a comment made by "Ramasini" to the effect that physicians, owing to the cheerfulness of their minds when they return with full pockets from visiting their patients, often escape free from epidemic diseases; they are never so much out of order as when nobody else is sick.[192]   (38a) The story of King David and Abishag the Shunamite is a case in point: "... they covered him with clothes, but he gat no heat. Wherefore his servants said unto him, let there be sought for my lord the king a young virgin ... that my lord the king may get heat."   (38b) The quotation in Greek given in Gaub, *tên parthenon synoikeein andri*, appears to be a paraphrase of Hippocrates, but the meaning is the same.   In a discussion of the states of anxiety seen in young girls, accompanied by bad dreams, unrestrained language and suicidal attempts, which the writer attributes to retention of the menses, the advice is given to marry them off as quickly as possible.[193]

XVIII   Corporeal Effects of Expressed and Suppressed Emotions Compared

39. I came now to the more violent emotions, those called forth by the thought of present or impending evil.   Other than to do no harm, they are rarely of benefit to the hale and hearty and may on occasion be injurious, but in the ill they sometimes work cures of

marvellous compass with unbelievable speed, of a kind that cannot be duplicated by any aids of the art whatsoever. You may wish, gentlemen, for me to demonstrate and prove this with facts, nor would I refuse but for a fear of being entangled by their abundance and continuing longer than your courtesy permits. Indeed, were I to search through my own store of observations and through the medical reports of past and present times such a large number of instances would present themselves that since all could not be brought forward I would be uncertain in choosing what best to mention or omit.

40. Striving for brevity, therefore, I wish you to understand first of all that in general the more abruptly an attack of an emotion breaks out the more violently and forcefully the whole man is shaken outwardly and within, and the greater is its weight to overthrow disease. Hence the less violent emotions, which attack without tumult and, once established, seat themselves in the pith and marrow as it were, to cause injury by hidden erosion rather than by open force, in the manner of grief, fear, hate, envy and the like, rarely if ever do anything beneficial for the body and are almost always harmful. Thus it is that anger and terror, the most destructive of the affections, display the greatest power in both directions and reveal themselves to be the most beneficial as well.

(39) We may conveniently list some eighteenth-century opinions on the general corporeal effects of the emotions at this point. Stahl states that the emotions may give rise to many diseases because of their power to direct and change various movements of the body. We are accustomed, he says, to quote Galen's statement that the characteristics of the mind are determined by those of the body, but, although emotional changes do arise from the disposition of the body and its humors, there is more truth in the converse.[194] The temperament of the body (meaning by this, Stahl writes,

the inter-relationships between its solid and fluid constituents) is frequently altered by the mind. While the order of emotions and tendencies impressed on the mind by heredity and custom cannot be completely inverted, nevertheless dominant emotions can be reduced to the second or third place by a contrary habit.[195] Valangin tells us that opposite emotions usually produce contrary effects on the body, hence one emotion may be the most suitable cure for the bodily effects of its opposite. The sympathy of the body and mind is, he says, such that particular affections of the mind will bring on particular disorders of the body, and disorders of the body will in turn affect the mind.[196] Boerhaave says that emotions may have effects precisely like those of certain corporeal stimuli.[197] A severe enough emotional disturbance may even lead to phthisis.[198] He asks us to consider that the interior of the body may be as greatly affected by emotional states as the exterior can easily be observed to be.[199] In my professional capacity, says Corp, I have often seen patients whose bodily complaints originated purely from a discomposed state of mind.[200] According to Zückert, all emotions have in common an alteration of the state of the body, and changes in the body and the mind can be reciprocally the causes or the effects of emotions.[201] Smith states that nothing produces more sudden or surprising changes in the body than violent affections of the mind. Horrible and unexpected sights, great grief, terror, anger and so forth will throw some people into hysterical convulsions, and in delicate women strong emotions may produce a peculiar state of immobility and partial insensibility.[202] Smith assimilates mental to nervous diseases and regards the "subtle medium" contained in the nerves as the bond between "two distinct substances, the soul and the body".[203] He claims that in almost every disease the nerves suffer more or less, and that there are few disorders which are not in some sense nervous. The complaints arising from weak or unnatural conditions of the nerves are so various that it is extremely difficult to describe or enumerate them. The nervous disturbance can mimic almost every ailment, and furthermore there are few chronic diseases with which such disturbances are not inter-mixed.[204] Boerhaave observes that violent or lasting emotions may fix and pervert the brain, nerves and muscles. Hence they are capable of causing or supporting many kinds of corporeal diseases.[205] Statements of this kind by clinical observers of the eighteenth century could be multi-plied almost without end. The opinions of some earlier writers may be found in the notes.[206, 207] (40) The point that violent emotional outbursts have potential therapeutic value, whereas suppressed emotions are almost always harm-ful, is more clearly stated by Gaub than by any of his con-temporaries.

XIX Anger as a Therapeutic Agent

41. Since anger arouses into activity everything in the body endowed with motive power and abruptly directs vital heat into every part by forcibly accelerating the movement of the blood—the story has been told that when Alexander the Great was in India he was once so furious that his body gave off glittering sparks of light—there is no reason to be surprised that while it incites certain acute and severe diseases and danger-ously worsens those already present, it may at times, when the harassed natural powers have become weakened by diseases of long duration, lead to an un-expected access of strength and an early recovery. According to Gellius a certain Samian athlete, enraged by the discovery that the drawing of lots in a sacred contest was not being carried out in good faith, spoke for the first time, and from then on spoke without stammering or difficulty for the rest of his life. A Frenchwoman lost her voice following delivery due to retention of the afterbirth. Mute for some time, she became angry in the course of a quarrel with her husband and tried to voice her protests; she spoke, indeed, and forthwith recovered the use of her tongue.

A certain Dane, in Borrichius, who had been deprived of his voice for four years, was similarly used by fortune. By chance meeting a little old woman whom he had long disliked he at once burst into abuse, his whole soul soon taking fire. Aware that he was speaking he regretted and deplored at the same time the ungodly auspices under which his voice had been restored. I myself recall an intermittent and very stubborn quartan fever converted by an outburst of anger into a continuous fever which, though not without danger, nevertheless in a short time expelled the unwelcome guest and was itself happily overcome. Willius mentions a hunter, so badly affected by severe arthritis that even in remissions of the pains he was unable to move about except four legged, supported by crutches, whom a certain well-known medical Hecuba convinced after a consultation that the whole trouble had been brought on by the charms and machinations of an old woman who lived nearby. Inflamed and completely infuriated by the desire for revenge he immediately went to the witch and having inflicted a thousand curses and blows on the miserable woman his misfortune was so well revenged that, while striking the blows, he felt the former vigor of his limbs return and his pains cease, and he returned home without crutches, never again to suffer from the same illness. An amazing cure indeed! What the art of medicine was quite unable to accomplish—to pluck out the joint disease by the roots —or could not accomplish except slowly and with a wealth of remedies and a sober way of life, the mind performed at one stroke, burning with anger and aided by violent motion of the body. I shall say more. Anger can recall to life those who are nearly dead. That Englishman of Robinson's, moribund and his pulse fading away, was revivified for the space of an hour after an attack of anger, with his powers resurgent and his pulse restored, but he rapidly expired as soon as his emotional disturbance was quieted.

(41a) Although Gaub seems to relate the Frenchwoman's loss of voice to retention of the afterbirth[208] we must not suppose that he considered this to be the sole cause of her condition, which he undoubtedly regarded as hysteria. The following paragraph mentions hysterical aphonia in the same connection. There were still survivals in Gaub's day of the Galenical belief that the organic basis of hysteria was retained, corrupted, "seed".[209] (41b) Gaub, of course, does not mean us to take the story of Alexander seriously.[210] (41c) The tale of the Samian athlete may be found in Gellius, where it is given without comment as to the cause of the restored power of speech together with the somewhat similar story of the son of Croesus (mentioned by Gaub in the following paragraph).[211] (41d) For other references in this paragraph see the notes.[212] (41f) Zückert believes that when anger is aroused the blood is driven with "unbelievable force" through various parts of the body, in particular the extremities,[213] and Corp holds that this is the cause for hemorrhages from the ears, nose, lungs, uterus and anus which may accompany anger.[214] Where Corp sees a resemblance between the effects of anger and those of excessive joy, Zückert sees one between anger and terror; in fact he calls anger a form of terror due to an injustice suffered.[215] Pechlin discusses the use of anger in the treatment of paralysis, gout and arthritis, but he warns his readers against the "new repute" of this "doubtful remedy". Even though Hippocrates permitted the use of terror, he says, one should have a very profound acquaintance with disease before trying it.[216] Corp tells of a paralytic who sprang from his chair in a fit of rage, and of a man who stammered except when he was angry. As for the reports that intermittent fevers, gout, and agues have been cured by the use of anger, Corp remarks that more often than not these diseases have been made more severe or even brought on by this emotion. The effects of anger are too transient and uncertain for physicians to employ it therapeutically; furthermore, the disease so treated may recur and become worse. "The ancients", he says, "seem to have considered anger as a remedy on the same principle they supposed a fever to be salutary; viz., by causing a concoction or resolution of viscid humors or by dispersing on the surface of the body those noxious matters which it had imbibed: hence it hath been imagined that the employment of anger would be useful, by enabling nature to expel the matter of small-pox, measles, erysipelas, and other eruptive diseases, from the internal and vital organs of the body. Experience, however, has taught us that in those disorders as they occur in this country such treatment would be highly injurious—placidity and calmness of mind being almost the first requisite to their happy termination".[217] Like Pechlin a century before him Corp says that "modern writers" cite Hippocrates as an authority for the employment of anger in the management of certain diseases, but he believes that they give too little attention to Hippocrates' caution that it should be employed if at all only in persons of "cold constitution".[218]

XX   Terror as a Therapeutic Agent

42. The healing virtue of terror, however, is both greater and more far-reaching, extending to even more kinds of disease. I shall not tarry here to set this forth as carefully and minutely as befits the topic, since instances of recoveries by this remedy are so well known and so numerous that I am quite confident that if I mention only a few each of you will at once recall many others encountered previously. What ancient tradition tells of the son of Croesus, King of Lydia—he was totally unable to talk even when almost full grown and uttered words for the first time when in fear and terror lest his father be killed by an invading foe—seems indeed like a miracle yet is not so unusual that it has not happened from that time on down to the present day, and I myself recall having many times seen hysterical patients who had lost the power to speak after an attack of their disease fully recover the use of their tongues when overcome by a sudden fright. It is well

established that mental aberrations of all kinds whatsoever, maniacal, hysterical, hypochondriacal and febrile, are often thus healed in a moment. A man in this city who was deranged by an acute fever immediately recovered from his delirium when he heard that his neighbor's house was in flames. A certain student at our university was so stricken by melancholy that he was sent home in desperation of his state; the ship in which he was borne violently collided with an oncoming ship in the darkness and, trembling all over from the unexpected collision, he promptly recovered. Shall I reckon up the maniacs recalled to sanity by terror, either intentionally arranged or occurring by chance? The hypochondriacs freed in a moment of the highly absurd fancies to which they had clung for so long? Chance first taught physicians that a headlong fall into the sea or submersion in water, employed in ancient times against rabies, is of great help against many such diseases, and this has been confirmed by experience. The inhabitants of Lyons showed Borrichius, during his travels in France, a lofty site from which the insane were thrown headlong into the Rhône and repeatedly drawn out on a line in order to teach them sense again, this measure having been adopted for its good results and not as a punishment. Helmont testifies that with this bold measure the English physician Robertson restored the use of reason to many insane persons. Why do I repeat what has already been said in my previous discussion? To the end, indeed, that you will understand, with regard to the point at issue, that the entire effect, great as it is, is not in the least due to some peculiar virtue of water but solely to the precipitation of the mind into the depths of terror and anguish as a result of the threat of suffocation. What is needed, then, is a machine that will inspire extreme terror, and submersion of such duration and frequency that life itself is put in hazard and doubt arises when the man is withdrawn whether he is quite dead or can still be revived; otherwise nothing fully effective is to be awaited. I pass over the intermittent fevers, in particular the deep-seated quartan that was the shame of medicine until the discovery of the effect of Peruvian bark, driven away by terror alone. That vigorous and celebrated army commander noted by Boyle, to his own benefit terrified by the sight of dormice although unafraid of everything else, after suffering for a long time from a stubborn quartan fever that responded to no remedy, not even to a change of climate, owed his recovery in the end to the unexpected assault of a dormouse. Rarely, as I have shown above, arthritis is relieved by anger, but frequently, however, by terror. Salmuth remarks a certain gouty patient whose hands and feet had been covered with poultices of milk, flour and turnips in order to relieve the pain. After the servants had left their master, a pig is said to have forced its way into the room through a door inadvertently left open. Attracted by the odor it began to devour the poultice, and the rough assault of the disorderly beast threw the man to the floor, not without the greatest emotional disturbance but with the result that his pains abated from then on and shortly thereafter entirely disappeared, never to return again. Many years ago when a terrible storm shook our city and the surrounding country, frightening the inhabitants and causing much damage everywhere, it had the happy effect on two invalids then in my care that with the help of terror one of them who had been deprived of the use of his feet for a long time by severe arthritis, was taught to flee unhelped from the imminent danger of a collapsing fireplace, and the other, contrary to my expectations, completely recovered from severe epilepsy. Moreover, I know of a man still alive on whom, as a boy, terror inflicted falling sickness, against which remedies were tried in vain; he too happily recovered a year later after another shock, the antidote no less than the poison drawn from the same source, just as people stung by scorpions are in the habit of seeking a remedy from the same creatures.

43. It is common knowledge that terror often checks hiccups, toothache, earache, headache and dangerous hemorrhages in a moment. And why should I not ascribe to the same source the fact that in past and present times many men overcome by sleep-inducing diseases, or deprived of their senses by fainting, taken for dead, placed on the bier, and even carried to the funeral pyre, have recovered life and sense due to the weeping and wailing of the bystanders, the sharp edge of the anatomist's knife, the clumsy joggling of the litter, or even the heat of the flames? Terror, however produced, is often the means by which the mind, as if aroused from slumber, quickly revivifies the dormant vital powers of the whole body.

(42a) Gaub's list of diseases known to have been cured as the result of terror[219] includes hysteria and hypochondria, two conditions which many medical writers regarded as variants of the same disease, following in the footsteps of the great seventeenth-century clinician Thomas Sydenham, the "English Hippocrates".[220] The importance of Sydenham's views on hysteria and hypochondriasis necessitate their presentation here. Besides equating the two afflictions Sydenham pointed out that the remote or external cause was most often a "mental disturbance", while the efficient, internal, immediate cause was a disorder of the nervous spirits giving rise to pain, spasm and functional disturbances. Both conditions were, ultimately, diseases of the nerves. However much ancient physicians have imputed hysteria to disease of the uterus, and modern physicians hypochondriasis to obstruction of the spleen or viscera, the two are alike as one egg is to another, Sydenham writes. It is true that women are more subject to the disease than men, but this has nothing to do with their anatomical peculiarities and is, rather, a consequence of a more sedentary mode of life. The multiformity of shapes which hysteria or hypochondriasis assumes is almost without limits. Hysteria is the Proteus, the chameleon of diseases; there is hardly any ailment that it may not mimic or part of the body that it may not affect, hence the unwary or unskilled physician is easily deceived into referring the symptoms to some essential disease of the bodily part seemingly affected. Seizures resembling genuine stroke, paroxysms resembling epilepsy, loin pain resembling renal colic due to stone, headache, vomiting, palpitations of the heart, convulsive coughing, diarrhea, localized transient swellings of the extremities, toothache and back pain are some of the many symptoms. One of the more characteristic findings is that "the patients at various times void a great quantity of limpid urine, clear as the water from the rock". In hypochondriasis of males and hysteria of females, according to Sydenham, this is an almost certain sign of the disease. Even a few seconds after passing water of the true straw-colored hue, a sudden and violent emotion may cause a man to produce an abundant flow of urine "of crystalline clearness". The frequency of hysteria is almost as remarkable as the variety of its symptoms. Sydenham says that it is the commonest of the chronic diseases, making up half their total. The acute diseases (chiefly fevers and their accompaniments) are, he writes, twice as common as the chronic diseases.[221] Half of all patients who are chronically ill, Sydenham is telling us, suffer from an ailment largely due to emotional disturbance. The therapy he proposes is a far cry from the "fair words" asked for by the Thracian physician mentioned in Plato's *Charmides*. It is a long list of drugs. (42b) Gaub does not discuss hysterical disorders either here or in his *Institutions*. We may presume that he shared the views of his age on the subject. A contemporary medical lexicon states that the uterus is falsely regarded as responsible for hysterical affections, whereas in reality the manifold symptom complex is the result of animal (i.e. psychological) or nervous and vital disturbances due to various diseases of the brain, heart, and uterus which themselves are the consequence of impurities in the blood and nervous fluid; on this subject see the Notes.[222]   The peculiar feature noted by Sydenham, the passage of large amounts of colorless urine in times of emotional stress, is also described by Boerhaave and related to the relaxation of muscular sphincters observed in emotional states in general.   Boerhaave comments that hysterical and hypochondriacal individuals are often forced to make more water in one day than they would otherwise in three— "colorless, odorless, and tasteless, like water flowing from a fountain".   This is due to relaxation of the muscular sphincters which determine the proportions between the arterial trunks and their branches.   In a similar way, Boerhaave adds, the emotions may disturb all passages in which the humors are prepared, transferred and eliminated; this is the reason why in a fit of rage one man vomits, another passes water, a third sweats, and a fourth defecates. Since all of the viscera, vessels and sphincters are involved, and since the velocity of motion (of the humors) is so altered, there is no doubt, Boerhaave says, that all bodily secretions and excretions can be disturbed by the emotions alone.[223] In Smith's discussions of the complaints arising "from unnatural conditions of the nerves" (where the condition here called hysteria is meant) he comments on the frequent discharge of large quantities of "limpid urine".[224]   While the cause of hysteria is "essentially established in the uterus", Laroque says obscurely, the chief (presumably remote) causes are emotional disturbances, *les passions de l'âme.* The uterus is provided with a great quantity of nerves, he points out, and its convulsions (excited by the emotional disturbance transmitted through the nerves) spread by sympathy to the head and chest and arouse a center of vitality which deprives the other parts of the body (of vital force). Hence vertigo, delirium and sluggishness.   Of help in the diagnosis of hysteria is the peculiar sensation often described by afflicted persons as if a ball were rising in their throats, cutting off respiration and threatening strangulation.[225] (42c) Gaub mentioned submersion therapy in the treatment of the insane in §95 of his first lecture.   There anxiety was held to produce the cure.   Here he calls for a machine to inspire terror. Whether he means an additional apparatus is not entirely clear, but probably he does not.[226] The Helmont referred to in the text is Franciscus Mercurius van Helmont (1618–1699, son of the more famous Jean Baptiste) who had stated that his father had observed recovery from mental disorders (due to emotional derangement) in afflicted persons "by chance falling into the water, and being taken up for dead". Dr. Richardson, he says (not Robertson), "recovered many" in this way.[227] (42d) In the previous paragraph Gaub told us of a patient whose intermittent quartan fever was converted into a more tractable form by an attack of anger. Now we are told of the cure of a quartan fever by terror. The reference to Peruvian bark, the source of quinine, indicates that the disease in question is malaria. Robert Boyle relates the story of the army commander who was "strangely fearful of rats" (not of dormice as Gaub says) together with an account of Salmuth's patient in a discussion of the therapeutic effects of the emotions.[228] Boyle accepted the medical doctrine of the non-naturals (whatever he may have thought of the term) as the following passage shows: "And thus (to be short) the passions of the mind such as fear, joy and grief, are given to man for his good, and, when rightly used, are very advantageous, if not absolutely necessary to him; though, when they grow unruly, or are ill-mannered, as it but too often happens, they frequently prove the causes of disease."[229] (43) Fear and terror may be effectively used in the treatment of melancholy, insanity, fevers, arthritis and paralysis, says Pechlin. He tells the story of a friend whose persistent tertian fever had resisted all treatment for four months but disappeared at once when he was in great fear of death.[230] Although Pechlin admits the effectiveness of terror in some cases of fever he calls it a "rustic and semibarbarous" method, perilous to apply and difficult to control.[231] The cure of hydrophobia by induced terror is another matter; its use here is permissible, especially when brought on by suddenly exposing the patient to the water he so much fears. Pechlin has also seen terror effectively used to check hemorrhage from the nose and uterus.[232] Stahl knows of a youth with "three-day fever" cured by fright occasioned by the sight of approaching soldiers. He mentions also the report of a paralyzed and bedridden man who recovered power of movement and escaped from his house when a fire broke out.[233] Boerhaave describes the remarkable therapeutic procedure in cases of mental disturbance of a certain practitioner in northern Holland (so successful that some of the highest men in the country were committed to his care). The patient is treated with the utmost consideration and his every wish granted, but the moment the disorder asserts itself he is seized and soundly beaten. Afterwards he is again treated with the utmost liberality and humanity, and given everything he wants; at last his fear of a beating is so great that he puts his madness aside. In this way cures have been wrought in "men of the highest dignity", so that after a few years they were able to "return to the service of the republic".[234] The use of submersion in the treatment of insanity is mentioned but recommended for the most desperate cases only.[235] Valangin warns that attempts to cure fever with terror are dangerous, since terror itself may induce convulsions.[236] Juncker attempts to account for certain "sympathetic" cures of macules and fleshy excrescences of the skin on the basis of the physiology of terror. He mentions the practice of touching the lesion with the hand of a corpse. Here the localized effect of terror is thought to cause a constriction of small blood-vessels and thus block the flow of the humors from which the lesion derives its nourishment.[237] Corp argues that the surprising strength shown by invalids when their lives or property are in danger, although commonly regarded as an immediate effect of terror, is produced rather by a strong desire to escape. However, he describes a patient of his own in whom the effects of fear on the urinary organs and "absorbent system" were most extraordinary. She was a fifty-five-year-old woman with ascites or dropsy of the belly. Corp warned her that the fluid must be withdrawn and the patient, although exceedingly apprehensive, consented to the procedure. Returning the next day Corp found that she had passed a large quantity of urine overnight, yet hardly more than a "large tea-cupful" per day had been passed for the preceding several weeks. Before the use of quinine, Corp recalls, terror was employed in the treatment of intermittent fevers and was induced by "hanging toads around the neck, or exposing the patient to other objects of dread".[238] Corp believed that the recurrence of certain intermittent diseases, especially those of the nervous system, was dependent on "the force of habit". Whatever interrupted this habit by affecting the brain or nervous system could prevent the recurrence of the disease. The return of the disorder was probably hindered by the high degree of attention that terror enforces, since "as in every other strong emotion or passion, the mind is wholly engaged by the object which excites it". With respect to a notable cure performed by Boerhaave, he suggests that the results would have been equally successful had the attention of the young patients been engaged in some other way than by terror.[239] Corp does not, in general, favor the use of fear. "In our day", he writes, "medical resources are sufficiently numerous to preclude the adventitious aid of terrific causes." The general tendency of fear is injurious, and it would be best to dispense with its use, since it can neither be directed or restrained.[240]

XXI   The Role of the Mind and the Emotions in the Cause and Cure of Bodily Disease

44. So much for this. My oration has traveled long enough in this vast sea of observations. It is now time to direct course where I aim, so that we may reach port as quickly as possible. I err, gentlemen! It only remains for you to understand that I have already made port. I am indeed convinced that the careful management of the mind, with which I have

undertaken to deal in this hour, is the concern of everyone and above all that of the physician, since it involves the health of the body, and that this may be derived with so little labor from the many and weighty arguments I have set forth that were I to undertake to demonstrate it with a great apparatus of words I would fear to annoy you or seem to distrust your abilities.   I have in addition certainly made it quite plain that the causes and occasions of a great many affections of the body arise in the mind, as it were from a fountainhead. It follows that not only do the healthy have a powerful garrison for the defense of their health in the properly managed activities of the mind, but also that good results are hardly to be obtained in treating the ill who suffer because of the guilt of the mind unless treatment is directed at the primary source of the evil, the mind itself.   I have stated further that the mind has many and very powerful resources against ill health, with which we may at times alleviate or cure diseases more surely or safely than with any other kind of remedy whatsoever.

(44) Gaub summarizes several points of his thesis here: (1) the causes and occasions of a great many affections of the body arise in the mind, (2) the mind can be a bulwark of bodily health, (3) in many cases of bodily disease treatment must be directed against the mind as the source of the bodily complaint, (4) bodily diseases may often be more readily alleviated or cured by the mind, that is, by the emotions, than by "corporeal remedies".   It was Gaub's stated intention in the second lecture to emphasize the controlling power of mind over body and to complete the discussion, initiated in the first lecture, of the "two occasions" on which the art of medicine is required to concern itself with the mind.

XXII   The Double Role of the Physician in Controlling the Mind for the Benefit of the Body

45. This being so, is there anyone who does not now see that the physician has a double role in controlling the mind for the benefit of the body—on the one hand to amend or ward off such causes of disease as are due to mental excess and on the other to relieve the ill by making good and skilful use of the mind's curative faculties?

46. There, stated in a few words, is the sum of our practice! Whoever knows how to search out these things with skill and act on them with care and foresight, to bring various things into harmony for the benefit of the different individual constitutions of all kinds of men whatsoever, the well and the ill, will in truth have attained the supreme peak of medical wisdom. But this is the heart of the difficulty! Hear the aphorism of the divine Hippocrates! "Life is short, the art long, occasion fleeting, experience treacherous and judgement difficult. Not only must he be prepared to do the necessary himself, but also to see that the patient, the attendants and the externals work together!"

XXIII   The Physician's Difficulties and Limitations

47. This is a wise and most worthy introduction to the practical aphorisms of a man supreme in the exercise of the art, comprehending with inimitable brevity the weightiest difficulties of the medical task of which I speak! I grant indeed that physicians, when they give instructions for the care and maintenance of the health, not only hold in general that the

management of the mind is most beneficial but also carefully expound one by one the effects of age, sex, temperament and manner of life, nor are they remiss in the task of explaining the harm that corrupt behavior inflicts on the life and health. Repeated and rammed down a thousand times this may keep men from profligacy, if only they are willing to learn. Therefore one might easily suppose that nothing is wanting on this side. But the truth is, unless everything deceives me, that anyone who is not content with mere theory and wishes to devote himself to the practice of medicine as well ought to believe quite otherwise. For the crux of the matter is to convert the knowledge of healing, which we have acquired through zeal and drudgery, into the fruit of public use. Indeed, since we have to care for the health of individual men it is not sufficient for us to consider only that which is common to the many but rather, and chiefly, that which is peculiar to each man, and here the differences are so great that in the entire race of man you will hardly find two who are exactly alike. It follows that the medical doctrine handed down for the benefit of the beginner is far more restricted in respect to the differences of men than the extent of the matter warrants, hence that the rules of life drawn from this doctrine admit of so many exceptions when applied to particular men that it becomes very difficult to establish anything for certain. And what shall I say of the tyranny of custom?—which not only forces mind and body into servitude but prescribes for physicians arbitrary rules in the care of both the well and the ill that must nevertheless be unwillingly obeyed or vainly opposed when contrary to the best maxims of the art. What of the prejudiced beliefs that are, as all know, so difficult to pluck out once deeply rooted? How often are we, after a fruitless struggle, forced in the end to deviate from the path of correct treatment, to omit what needs to be done, to permit what we would prefer to forbid, or to alter in some other way a prudently designed course of action? Let us nevertheless suppose, gentlemen, what is most uncommon, that none of all these things that make for difficulties and hindrances obtain! Who is so lynx-eyed and so experienced and capable that he can foresee and ward off or moderate the difficulties coming from without, whether they occur by chance or are caused by bystanders? Countless such things happen every day and they are very often of such importance that for no other reason the well grow ill and the ill grow worse and succumb to disease, and the physician certainly does not have the power to relieve them. For it is indeed primarily from this source that emotional disturbances, those deadly pests of mankind, arise, through which most of the circumstances that I have just mentioned introduce poison into the bodily economy. Hence the manifold insults to the health, hence the antecedent causes and provocations of so many diseases, and the host of difficulties, hindrances and disappointments in treatment, all of which would indeed not vex the physician if it were within the power of the art to ward off at will the impending tumults of the mind or to repress and calm those that had already broken out. Since we know from experience that neither sound reason, moral doctrine nor religion itself can effectively counter them, compassion sometimes makes us silently regret that man is denied the power of altering circumstances as need requires, nor can he always produce from the pharmacopeia a sure means for affording relief to a body troubled by an unquiet mind. When the courtier who has lost the favor of his prince, the merchant suddenly reduced to extremity by misfortune, the mother in desperation after the sad death of her husband or only child, are unable to bear the burden of unhappiness with equanimity and fall ill in body in consequence of distress of mind, how much more rapidly and surely could they be relieved if the physician were able to make good the loss they lament! The madness of the first king of Judea could indeed be allayed but not extinguished, since the judgement of God was irrevocable, by the harp of David. Nor is it likely that Perdiccas and Antiochus, whom I mentioned above, would have otherwise shaken off their lethargy had the authority of the physicians been insufficient to permit the quenching of their desires. Although these disastrous external events are for the most part not to be altered, nevertheless whenever such as admit of some degree of moderation take place the physician is required to leave untried nothing that can properly be done to preserve, or restore when upset, the tranquillity of mind of those who are committed to his care. And so, to the practice of the art which is sufficiently burdened by its own difficulties, the greater difficulty that we cannot therefore always avoid being involved in other people's affairs is added, and even with the most careful management this is rarely accomplished so happily that the thanks obtained equal the troubles endured.

(47a) Gaub's opening remarks indicate that physicians were accustomed (in keeping with the doctrine of the non-naturals) to explain to their patients the harmful and beneficial effects of the emotions on bodily health. But, he says, the exhortation and advice of the physician is often useless in the face of his inability to foresee, prevent or redress the difficulties arising from without that are the source of emotional disturbances. If the physician could produce from the pharmacopeia relief for a "body troubled by an unquiet mind", the situation would be improved, Gaub remarks, returning again to the chief thesis of his first lecture. Since the physician is as a rule unable to influence the external circumstances causing his patient's emotional disturbance, only this remains. When it lies within his power to control the external circumstances for the benefit of his patient the physician should do so. Gaub, however, finds that the physician's difficulties are sufficiently great without further involvement in his patient's private life. (47b) Gaub mentioned loss of favor at court as one of the misfortunes that might lead to bodily disease. The condition bore the name of *Hofkrankheit* (*mal de cour*) and is often mentioned with the closely related condition known as *Damenkrankheit* (*maladie des dames à quarante ans*), both being largely due to the effects of grief in the opinion of eighteenth-century medical writers. Weikard, for example, calls *Hofkrankheit* a gnawing evil due to a mixture of covetousness, envy and grief. When the currying of favor at court is the goal of all efforts the courtier becomes peevish and morose if he is not accorded his customary distinction, and he may fall physically ill if the countenance of his sovereign turns away from him. The English ambassador at Petersburg once remarked, according to Weikard, "*à Petersbourg il n'y a que deux maladies, les hémorrhoïdes et le mal de cour*". The sufferer loses cheerfulness, appetite and color. Cicero and Seneca labored under this disease and in every region and in every class of society we may observe something analogous to *Hofkrankheit*, Weikard comments.[241] The *maladie des dames à quarante ans* is similar to *Hofkrankheit*. What is due in one to loss of favor at court is due in the other to the loss of beauty and suitors.[242] Boerhaave mentions that the loss of a king's favor may literally mean death to a man of the court.[243]

XXIV   The Physician Must Attempt to Control the Mind Through the Body, But He Should not Wholly Suppress the Emotions

48. With such difficulty in controlling the events which strike men down, the only thing remaining for the physician is to direct his attention to the management of the mind itself, and strive with all zeal and effort to learn to restrain, moderate and bring to order

that principle of arousal, the *enormôn*, whose vehemence leads the thwarted mind of man astray to the detriment of his body. Yet do not consider me an adherent of the Stoic sect, gentlemen, one who either expects or wishes to induce in men's minds by means of medical procedures the "impassivity" that the philosopher Zeno vainly attempted to inculcate with his doctrines. So far is this from my belief that I fully agree with what Gellius states Herodes Atticus said against the Stoics with regard to the matter, that the disposition grows far too torpid and inactive when it is deprived of the support of the affections, and that the proponents of "impassivity" are like the Thracian who knew nothing of farming: when he happened to see his neighbor cleaning out brambles and pruning the vines, olives and trees in order to get a richer and more fruitful crop he stupidly mutilated in imitation all of the vines and olives on his own land, cutting off the sprouts, branches and foliage of the trees and plucking out the fruit-bearing shrubs and bushes along with the thorns, only to be taught in the end by the bad results that to cut everything down indiscriminately is not the same as to remove carefully what interferes with the harvest. Nor does only the mind gradually succumb to lethargy, for this emptiness of the affections leads also to a weakening of the circuit of the humors, the bodily impetus slackening in harmony so that finally the vigor of life itself is sapped. Thus it happens, as I have shown above, that in emotions of violent nature there are medicinal as well as harmful powers, of tremendous help in the relief of ailments, so that physicians should not wish for men to do without them entirely.

(48a) Once again Gaub shifts back to the theme of his first lecture. The physician finds himself forced to manage the mind indirectly, by means of agents acting on the body. But he must avoid inducing the *apatheia* of the Stoics, since the emotions are essential to the health of both body and mind.   (48b) Gaub refers here to Gellius and quotes almost verbatim a passage citing Herodes Atticus.[244]

XXV   The Role of the Physician in Managing the Whole Man

49. It would therefore seem that the greatest pains should be taken to have this disorderly part of the mind under the control of the judgement at all times, to check its activities when they are about to erupt, to moderate them when they exceed due measure, and to arouse and direct them to any extent whatsoever that circumstances require.   I do not indeed deny that this matter has been discussed no less fully than clearly by both ancient and modern philosophers, so that it may therefore seem to some strange for me to want something more ample and complete, and to propose that the physician work out what is properly the business of the philosopher.   But, although I praise and approve of the maxims of the philosophers having to do with the control of the emotions, and freely admit that they are not without all value in medical practice—for in friendly conversation and cheerful words, in serious discussions and stern warnings, in convincing predictions and threats, there is a kind of power that allows one to control the emotions at will, as if with whip and reins, when their proper use is understood—they recommend themselves for the most part more in theory than in use.   Anyone can easily see that they are not applicable to all times, places and persons, nor is it given to everyone to apply them wisely and prudently, since they are drawn out of that spring of sound reason from which few can command much, and very often they fail even when rightly applied; we know from experience that even the more cultivated spirits do not always hit the mark.   After Dionysius of

Herakleon had spent many years teaching himself fortitude with the aid of Zeno's philosophy he was forced in the end to cry out and lament the falsity of what he had hitherto thought of pain when suffering from a pain in the kidneys. The violence and inflexibility of these disturbances is sometimes so great that they prevent all use of reason, and whoever desires to govern them by precept will finally recognize in frustration what he might already have learned from the comic poets, that he does no more than give himself the task of reasoning with unreason. It is known on the strength of observation that the sudden and unexpected—whereby the emotions usually exert their greatest effect on the body—when harmful, cannot be warded off by measures of this kind, and, when helpful, is for the most part more effectively induced by pure chance than by diligent activity.

50. Since in a matter of such importance nothing ought to be overlooked, I do not indeed wish to slight or disparage the supportive measures proffered by philosophers when of help. But if they have truly offered little of certain effect, this is no reason for the physician to lose hope, provided that he rightly understands the benefits to be derived from the storehouse of his own art. I refer, of course, to the management of the mind by means of the body, as set forth in my previous discussion. I believe that I then showed sufficiently well that the mind is bent in one direction or the other in accordance with the changing state of the body. When we cannot fully rely on the power of reason to control the emotions, and hence cannot govern the mind by means of the mind itself, the wealth of our art is such that we have many measures available which act at first on the bodily parts and movements only, yet these same effects act equally on the mind, the inhabitant of the body, and can, as with bit and spurs, restrain the overhasty or rouse and stimulate the sluggish.

51. You will observe, gentlemen, that both aspects of the management of the mind that I have said were the concern of the physician are linked together by a certain natural bond, and that one is weakened when deprived of the aid of the other. The course of the argument itself has gradually led me back to my starting point. It is now quite plain that mind and body, by virtue of their mutual relationship, lead a life in common with one another. When united in man their powers are so intimately compounded that whatever of good or bad, whether through chance or design, happens to one of the partners affects the other as well. Since I have already discussed this topic at length there is no reason for me to burden your ears, already excessively wearied by a prolonged oration, with further repetition.

(49) The *Tusculan Disputations* are cited in the text as the source of the story of Diomysius.[245] (50) In §98 of the first lecture Gaub called for the development of "special regimens, universal therapeutic methods, and particular remedies . . . by means of which we can awaken, sharpen or strengthen any faculty of the mind whatsoever, and can moderate, arouse, or repress its paroxysms, instincts and propensities as needed". Here he once again states the Galenical thesis that the mind is bent in accordance with the physical condition of the body, and calls upon the physician to become better acquainted with the therapeutic agents to be found in the storehouse of the medical art. (51) The final paragraph restates the unity of mind and body and we recall that in the first lecture Gaub said that mind and body were abstractions, made for the convenience of the physician who in the practice of his art always dealt with man as he is, an indissoluble union of both, the whole man.

Notes

Essay of 1747

1. Cicero's words are "...*etenim omnes artes, quae ad humanitatem pertinent, habent quoddam commune vinculum et quasi cognatione inter se continentur.* Gaub writes, similarly, "...*multae sunt...*, *quarum materies homo est artes atque scientiae...habent tamen omnes et singulae commune quoddam vinculum et quasi cognatione quadam inter se continentur...*" (*Cicero, The Speeches, with an English translation by N. H. Watts*, London, 1923, *Pro Archia*, I).

2. Jerome Gaub, *Institutiones Pathologiae Medicinalis, ed. alt.*, Leiden, 1775, §99. The most outstanding difference between a living organism and a lump of matter, it would seem, is that the former is a whole integrated in such a way that when one part is affected some or all of the other parts suffer in common. This is the literal meaning of "sympathy" (*sympatheia*), the term used by Stoic philosophers to designate a relationship of the kind exemplified by the living body. "Consensus" has a related, if not identical meaning in this context. Stoicism did not separate mind and body in an absolute, Cartesian, sense. Hence the Stoic philosophers were able to regard the *psyché* as the highest form of binding principle responsible for this dynamic state of union of parts characteristic of the living being, of which *physis* and *hexis* were the corresponding principles with respect to organic and inorganic structure. For a valuable discussion of Stoic views see S. Sambursky, *The Physics of the Stoics*, New York, 1959, especially Chap. I, "The Dynamic Continuum". The reaction of the whole organism to the injury of any one of its parts was clearly the archetype, so to speak, of these philosophical ideas. Heraclitus expressed this form of unity and sympathy in a striking comparison: the *psyché* is like a spider and the body like its web. The spider, sitting in the middle of her net, becomes aware that a fly has damaged a thread; she hurries to the spot as if the rupture had caused her pain; just so the *psyché* hurries to the site of a wound or injury, as if suffering herself (Hermann Diels, *Die Fragmente der Vorsokratiker, Griechisch und Deutsch, 7te Aufl., hrsg. W. Kranz*, Berlin, 1954, 3 vols., vol. 1, p. 166).

3. *Spiritus intus alit: totamque infusa per artus/mens agitat molem et magno se corpore miscet* (*Aeneid* VI, 726–27). On the Stoic treatment of the very important problem of mixture (*krasis*) Sambursky may be consulted (S. Sambursky, pp. 11–17). The Stoics distinguished mechanical mixture (mosaic-like mixture) from "fusion" leading to the formation of a new substance (corresponding to what would today be called a

chemical compound). Between the two lay a third case of mixture (*krasis* for liquids and *mixis* for non-liquids) in which complete inter-penetration of the components occurred, so that any smallest volume of the mixture was occupied by all components in the same proportion, each component preserving its own properties (as was not the case in fusion). In Stoic theory a material *pneuma* (and the *psychê* was looked on as a kind of *pneuma*) permeated the body in this third fashion and gave it its unity. Gaub has discarded the material *psychê*, but retained the other Stoic notions.

4. "...*ubicunque mens est corpus est*; *mens ubi corpus*...". This is very close to the third type of "mixture" mentioned in Note 3. With respect to the location of the mind, we must not forget that Descartes himself held that the mind was joined to the whole body and could not be said to be in one place to the exclusion of others (Descartes, *Œuvres et Lettres*, Librairie Gallimard, Paris, 1953, *Les Passions de l'Âme*, art. 30, p. 710). Descartes believed that the site where the mind chiefly exercised its control over the body was the pineal gland, but we must not confuse the location of mind with its site of action, as is often done. Koestler, for example, writes that Descartes housed the realm of the mind "in a somewhat niggardly fashion in the pituitary [sic] gland" (Arthur Koestler, *The Sleepwalkers*, New York, 1959, reprinted 1963, p. 525) and Arnold seems to suppose that Descartes believed that the "soul resides in the pineal gland" (Magda Arnold, *Emotion and Personality*, New York, 1960, 2 vols., vol. 1, p. 100).

5. Galen, *Opera Omnia*, ed. C. G. Kühn, Leipzig, 1821–33, vol. IV, pp. 767–822, *Hoti ta tês psychês êthê tais tou sômatos krasesin hepetai: Quod animi mores corporis temperamenta sequantur;* German translation by Erika Hauke, "Dass die Vermögen der Seele eine Folge der Mischun-gen des Körpers sind (*Hoti tais tou sômatos krasesin hai tês psychês dynameis hepontai*)", *Abhandlung zur Geschichte der Medizin und Naturwissenschaften*, Heft 21, Berlin, 1937; French translation by Charles H. Daremberg, "Que les mœurs de l'âme sont la conséquence des tempéraments du corps", *Œuvres de Galien*, 2 vols., Paris, 1854, vol. 1, pp. 47–91. Daremberg's extensive notes on this essay are well worth consulting in connection with Galen's claim that the *psychê* is material. He finds that Galen has misunderstood the Aristotelian doctrine of form and matter by failing to recognize that these two principles are primitive and co-equal (loc. cit., p. 54). See also Chauvet, who points to the contradictions in Galen's writings on the subject of the *psychê*, and makes the interesting remark that in reducing the *psychê* to the status of a modification of the body Galen expresses himself as a physician, while in regarding the *psychê* as a force which thinks and lives in the body by means of the organs he expresses himself as a philosopher (Emmanuel Chauvet, *La philosophie des médecins grecs*, Paris, 1886, pp. 286–302).

6. Celsus, *De medicina*, with an English translation by W. G. Spencer, London, 1948, 3 vols., vol. I, p. 5. Gaub's citation reads *A. Corn. Cels. Lib. I. praefat.* It was the opinion of Celsus that the healing art was most necessary to those whose bodily strength had been weakened by continual thought and restless vigils.

7. "*. . . quam quod suus quemque animus in semet ipsum atque in corpus suum reflexus quotidie, nec obscure, edocere possit*". See also Note 18.

8. Gaub uses the phrase *domicilium mentis*. More commonly the body has been called the home of the soul, *domicilium animae*, ". . . her house, abode, and stay", as Robert Burton says (*Anatomy of Melancholy*, 16th ed., London, 1836, Pt. 1, Sec. 2, Mem. 5, Subs. 1, p. 246).

9. Hence the pun, *sôma = sêma* in *Cratylus* 400. Some say that the body (*sôma*) is the grave (*sêma*), Socrates remarks, and the Orphic poets were under the impression that the body was a prison in which the psyche was incarcerated.

10. *Cratylus* 400, *Phaedrus* 250.

11. Gaub speaks of the "*inclusus detentusque animus*" and Cicero of the "*animus . . . in corpore inclusus* (*Tusculan Disputations, with an English translation by J. F. King*, Loeb Library, 1960, I, xxiv).

12. See L. J. Rather, "G. E. Stahl's Psychological Physiology", *Bull. Hist. Med.*, Baltimore, 35: 37–49, 1961.

13. "*Figurez-vous deux horloges ou deux montres, qui s'accordent parfaitement*", and later, "*Mettez maintenant l'âme et le corps à la place de ces deux horloges* ("Troisième éclaircissement. Extrait d'un lettre de Mr. Leibniz", *Journal des Savans*, 19 Nov., 1696, p. 452. *Leibn. Opp. ed. Dutens, Tom. II, P. 1*, p. 94, reprinted in Gottfried Wilhelm Leibniz, *Opera philosophica quae exstant latina gallica germanica*, 1959, Scientia, Aalen, 1959, p. 135).

14. "*. . . avec tant d'art et de justice, qu'on se puisse assurer de leur accord dans la suite; et c'est la voye de consentement préétablie* (Leibniz, *Opera philosophica*, p. 135).

15. "*. . . ad ipsam uniuscujusque vestrum conscientiam*". See also Note 18.

16. "*. . . non seulement la même quantité de la force totale des corps, qui ont commerce entre eux, mais encore leur direction . . .* (G. W. Leibniz, "Considérations sur le principe de vie et sur les natures plastiques par l'auteur de l'harmonie préétablie", *Histoire des Ouvrages des Savans, Mai 1705*, reprinted in *Opera philosophica*, pp. 429–30).

17. David Hume, *An Enquiry Concerning Human Understanding*, reprint of posthumous edition of 1777, La Salle, 1952, pp. 70–1 (Sect. VII, Pt. I).

18. For a discussion of the philosophical questions at issue here see Philip P. Hallie's *Maine de Biran, Reformer of Empiricism 1766–1824*, Cambridge, 1959, pp. 84–104. Hallie regards the central contribution of Biran to be his description and evaluation of man's internal experience of voluntary movement. Internal experience, for Biran, is its own

guarantee of truth, and Hume's difficulty arose from the confusion of two different realms of experience or knowledge.

19. "*Neque ut novam aliquam, quae magis congrua videatur, similitudinem comminiscar, hacque exornem, quod explicare non liceat*".

20. "*. . . omnia quae in homine sic fiunt, ut cogitatione in se habeant*" pertains to the mind, while "*. . . ea contra, in quibus motus aut ceterarum, quae naturam corpoream finiunt, proprietatum aliquid inest*" pertains to the body.

21. Gaub nowhere attempts to introduce surreptitiously an entity or function designed to overcome the philosophical difficulty inherent in the mind-body problem, e.g. von Hartmann's "rotation of molecules" (Eduard von Hartmann, *Philosophy of the Unconscious, translation of the 9th edition of 1884*, London, 1931, p. 170) or Eccles's "spatio-temporal field of influence" (John Eccles, *The Neurophysiological Basis of Mind*, Oxford, 1953, p. 272).

22. "*. . . par le nom de pensée, je comprends tout de qui est tellement en nous, que nous en sommes immédiatement connaissants . . . toutes les opérations de la volonté, de l'entendement, de l'imagination et des sens* (Descartes, *Réponses de l'auteur aux secondes objections recueillies de plusieurs théologiens et philosophes par le R. P. Mersenne*, p. 390).

23. "*. . . duo etiam sunt functionum hominis ordines*".

24. "*. . . quae medicis vitales atque naturales audiunt*". This division corresponds to the tripartite Galenical classification of the faculties and spirits: Galen's *pneuma physikon, pneuma zôotikon* and *pneuma psychikon* are the *spiritus naturalis, spiritus vitalis* and *spiritus animalis* of the Latin medical writers, i.e. the natural, vital and animal spirits ("animal", from *anima = psychê*, refers to the higher functions including those of volition and awareness).

25. Cicero, *Tusculan Disputations*, II, xx, xxi.

26. "*. . . auparavant garanti par la défense ou par la fuite contre les choses nuisibles*" (Descartes, *Les Passions de l'Âme*, §36, 38, pp. 713–14). The "fight or flight" antithesis is usually associated with the name of Walter Cannon. See *The Wisdom of the Body*, revised and enlarged edition 1939, reprinted 1963, New York, p. 227.

27. Descartes, *Traité de l'Homme*, p. 823–4. Descartes describes how his machine man withdraws its hand from the fire without participation of mind: a nerve impulse from the burnt part to the brain opens a tiny conduit and animal spirits flow to the muscles, causing withdrawal of the burnt part, turning of the eyes, and so on. Afferent and efferent paths are not fully described nor does the arc have a center in the spinal cord, but the principle of reflex movement is clearly set forth.

28. See Note 26.

29. "*Pulchram vero voluntatem! quam nisi extra mentem posuerint . . .*".

30. Descartes, *Les Passions de l'Âme*, §47, p. 718. See also Gaub II, 5 and commentary.

31. Gaub's phrase *"in ipsa morte"* suggests that he may have taken the episode from Montaigne, although the original source is Seneca's *De tranquillitate animi*, cap. xiv. In recounting the story Montaigne writes that "Canius Julius" had philosophized even in death, or at the point of death, itself: *"Cette-cy philosophe non seulement jusqu'à la mort, mais en la mort mesme"* (Montaigne, *Essais, texte établi et annoté par Albert Thibaudet*, Paris, 1950, ii/6, p. 407). (Gaub cites Montaigne in his second lecture, §21.)

32. *". . . hypochondria philosophi spissato humore obstruere"* . . . and *". . . in corpore ejus excitare causas anxietatis . . ."*.

33. *". . . morbi cohaerentiae in humoribus . . ."* (Gaub, *Institutiones*, §271, p. 94).

34. Ibid.

35. *". . . sensationes molestae ex morbo . . ."* (Gaub, *Institutiones*, §669–691, pp. 262–72).

36. Ibid., *". . . sentire mentem dicimus, cum ex corporis sui affectiones ideas concipit . . ."* (Gaub repeats here that the problem of how this can come about, given the radical difference in nature of body and mind, is not the concern of the physician).

37. Ibid.

38. Ibid. *"Anxietas, idcirco tristis quidem pariter ac dolore, sensatio est . . . longe terribilior, ipsa quandoque morte intolerabilior."*

39. Ibid.

40. *". . . quod utrum incitans, an impetum faciens, an cum Hippocrate enormôn an hormên, aut impetum et incitationem ipsam . . ."*.

41. Robert Boyle, for example, quotes with approval the "sober admonition" of Galen not to dispute about words when matters of fact are at stake, *cum de re constat, de verbis non est litigandum* (*The Sceptical Chymist*, 1661, reprinted London, 1949, Prop. IV, p. 34).

42. *". . . non bruta homo machina est . . . Mens intus est"* (Gaub, *Institutiones*, §99).

43. *". . . le contenant, le mouvant, le contenu . . ."* (Émile Littré, *Œuvres Complètes d'Hippocrate*, Paris, 1849, réimpression Amsterdam, 1962, ten vols., vol. 5, p. 347).

44. *". . . ea quae impetum faciunt . . ."* (Galen/Kühn, vol. XIV, p. 697).

45. *"Quidni praeeuntem sequamur Hippocratem? qui praeter continentia et contenta, etiam ta ormônta in homine contemplaci cum ratione jussit"* (Gaub, *Institutiones*, §188).

46. *". . . omnis perturbatio sit animi motus vel rationis expers vel rationem aspernans vel ratione non obediens, isque motus aut boni, aut mali opinione citetur"* (Cicero, *Tusculan Disputations*, III, xi).

47. *". . . non modo a perceptione simplici incipiant, sed insuper accedentem exigant boni aut mali, quod in oblata re esse videatur, repraesentionem . . ."*.

48. William McDougall, *Body and Mind*, 1911, reprinted 1961, Boston, p. 268.

49. A. E. Taylor, *A Commentary on Plato's Timaeus*, Oxford, 1928, p. 260.

50. Friedrich Ueberweg, *Die Philosophie des Altertums, herausgegeben von Karl Praechter, 12te Auflage*, Basel/Stuttgart, 1960, p. 480. See also Gaub II, §5 and commentary.

51. Magda Arnold states that psychologists have in the past analyzed the sequence emotion–expression–action, rather than the sequence perception–appraisal–emotion. She argues that the "felt emotion" cannot be identical with the "physical disturbance" because the felt tendency to approach or withdraw comes on immediately while the physical disturbance takes time to develop. Her definition of an emotion is as follows: a felt tendency toward or away from anything intuitively appraised and beneficial or harmful, respectively, together with physiological changes organized toward approach or withdrawal (Arnold, pp. 178–82). Arnold rejects Cartesian dualism but is unaware of her own, although it is the same in principle, since the fundamental problem of the relation of "raw feels" to neurophysiological states remains (cf. Herbert Feigl, *The "Mental" and the "Physical"*, in *Concepts, Theories, and the Mind–Body Problem*, vol. II, University of Minnesota, 1958, p. 372).

52. Gaub, *Institutiones*, §648.

53. Rudolf Virchow, "The Place of Pathology among the Biological Sciences", in *Disease, Life and Man*, selected essays by Rudolf Virchow, translated by L. J. Rather, Stanford, 1958.

54. "*. . . nervorum ista compages suo intus motore haud minus animatur, quam ipsa reliquam corporis molem, per quam diffusa est, agitat . . .*".

55. "*. . . duobus inter se distinctis constet systematibus . . .*".

56. "*. . . proxenata dici potest, cujus interventu mens atque organa corporis inter se communicant*".

57. "*. . . motionis principia . . .*".

58. Winslow in 1732 first used the term "sympathetic nerves" to designate those which had hitherto been designated "intercostal nerves". He described the chain of nervous ganglia lying adjacent to the spinal cord, calling them "little brains" (*petits cerveaux*), and observed their communications with the vertebral nerves. He suggested that the term "great sympathetic nerves" was suitable because of their numerous communications with other principal nerves of the body (Jaques-Benigne Winslow, *Exposition anatomique de la structure du corps humain. Nouvelle édition*, Amsterdam, 1743, vol. 3, pp. 218–34).

59. Gaub does not mention the pineal body whose movements, according to Descartes, directed the flow of animal spirits in the nerves. He was perhaps familiar with Winslow's discussion of this point and demonstration that the anatomical position of the gland made such movement impossible (Winslow, vol. 4, p. 216).

60. "*. . . potest igitur medicus cogitatione quidem illud ab animo abstrahere, atque seorsum contemplari; ut idearum compositione minus confundatur . . .*".

61. "...*cum homine, ut est, rem habet*...".
62. Gaub, *Institutiones*, §36, 39.
63. "...*ut illa posita, hic ponatur, durante duret, mutata mutetur, ablata tolletur*" (Gaub, *Institutiones*, §61). The distinction between practical and theoretical causes in medical thought has been brought out by R. G. Collingwood, who finds that in medicine a statement about the cause of a disease amounts to a statement about the way in which that disease should be treated. Two persons who treat the same disease in two different ways will make correspondingly different statements as to its cause. If the disease is somatic, but psychological treatment is nevertheless found helpful, a definition of its cause in psychological terms does not, according to Collingwood, imply a theory of interaction between two entities, body and mind, but merely restates the fact that psychological treatment has been found helpful (*Metaphysics*, Oxford, 1940, p. 306).
64. A little more than a century earlier Robert Burton had discussed the offices of the physician and the divine, the sum of whose efforts, he held, yields the "whole physician"; "It is a disease of the soul on which I am to treat and as much appertaining to a divine as to a physician ... one amends *animam per corpus* (soul through body) and the *corpus per animam* (body through soul) as our Regius Professor of physick well informed us in a learned lecture of his not long since. One helps the vices and passions of the soul, anger, lust, desperation, pride, presumption, etc. by applying that spiritual physick, as the other uses proper remedies in bodily diseases. Now this (the disease, melancholy) being a common infirmity of body and soul, and such a one that hath as much need of spiritual as a corporeal cure, I could not find a fitter task to busy myself about, a more apposite theme ... that should so equally participate of both, and require a whole physician" (*Anatomy of Melancholy*, p. 15). At about the same time we find Thomas Wright recommending his book, *The Passions of the Minde in Generall* (London, 1621) to "the Divine, the Philosopher, the curers both of the body and the soule, I meane the Preacher and the Physition" (loc. cit., p. 2). For the content of Wright's book see Notes II, 206.
65. "...*nostra arare vitula, cum parum forte sua profecerint*...".
66. The citation reads *Dissertat. de Methodo n. VI. p. m. 38* and the quotation is as follows: *Animum adeo a temperamento et organorum corporis dispositione pendere, ut si ratio aliqua possit inveniri, quae homines sapientiores et ingeniosiores reddat quam hactenus fuerunt, credendum sit illam in medicina quaeri debere.* Descartes's *Le Discours de la Méthode* was first published in French and the passage in question reads: *car même l'esprit dépend si fort du tempérament et de la disposition des organes du corps, que s'il est possible de trouver quelque moyen qui rende communément les hommes plus sages et plus habiles qu'ils n'ont été jusqu'ici, je crois que c'est dans la médecine qu'on doit le chercher* (Descartes,

pp. 168–9). Whether or not Descartes was aware of Galen's essay on moral behavior and bodily temperament is uncertain. Descartes was not in the habit of calling attention to his sources, as Leibniz remarked on one occasion (... *Mr. Descartes a usé d'artifice, pour profiter des descouvertes autres sans leur en vouloir paroitre redevable*. Leibniz, p. 142). The claim that medicine rather than philosophy holds the key to the understanding of the nature of man appears for perhaps the first time in a polemical essay, "On Ancient Medicine", part of the Hippocratic corpus. The writer rejects the views of the sophists, holding that medicine alone is the source of positive knowledge with respect to man (Hippocrates/Littré, 1, p. 261).

67. Ludwig Edelstein remarks that when Juvenal's "*mens sana in corpore sano*" is quoted the first three words "*orandum ut sit*" are usually omitted. But what Juvenal means, he says, is simply "let us pray that there be a sound mind in a sound body", not that only in a sound body could there dwell a sound mind. No ancient philosopher or physician, Edelstein claims, would assert that a sound body guarantees a sound mind, and Galen expressly denies that the dependence of the mind on the temperament of the body makes praise or blame of human actions superfluous ("The Relations of Ancient Philosophy to Medicine", *Bull. Hist. Med.*, 27: 299, 1952). Cf. Gaub I, 83.

68. Gaub, *Institutiones*, §14–16.

69. Ibid., §420. Gaub's words are "... *vocari medicis solent res non naturales, quasi tu dicas res medias, quae ex se, nec secundum, nec contra naturam sint, nec salubres, nec noxiae, at usu vel abusu tales fieri queant.*" Actually, the reason why they are called non-naturals is quite unclear, and Gaub's remark that the term indicates their position midway between things in accord with nature (*secundum naturam*) and against nature (*contra naturam*) has no real basis. (See Note 71. See also Introduction and Gaub II, 34c.)

70. *mens, corpus, res externae*, Ibid., §420.

71. Galen/Kühn, I, pp. 305–412, *Ars medica (Technê iatrikê)* contains the relevant passages. Medicine is the science of (1) the wholesome (or healthy), (2) the unwholesome, (3) that which is neither. Each of these is considered in turn under three headings: body, cause and sign. Further, causes are said to fall into two classes, (1) efficient and (2) conserving (loc. cit., p. 307). The conserving causes (*phylaktika aitia*) of health and disease include both necessary and non-necessary factors, the former being those which cannot be avoided and therefore the more important. They are numbered by Galen as follows: (1) air, (2) motion and rest, (3) sleeping and waking, (4) that which is taken in, (5) that which is excreted or retained, (6) the emotions or passions. Whether they are good or bad for the health depends on their various relations with other things (ibid., pp. 367–9). Turning to the Latin version of ibn Isḥāq's introduction to this book of Galen (Joannitius,

Isagoge ad tegni Galeni, Leipzig, 1497) we find that medicine is said to comprise the study of *rerum naturalium, non-naturalium* and of those which are *contra naturam*. The six "non-naturals" are then given as (1) *de mutatione aeris*, (2) *de modis ciborum*, (3) *de modis potationum*, (4) *de somno*, (5) *de coitu*, and (6) *de accidentibus animae*. In the Latin version of Avicenna's Canon, on the other hand, the *res non-naturales* appear among the efficient causes of disease (*Avicennae, liber canonis ... a Gerardo Carmonensi ex arabico sermone in latinum conversa*, Venice, 1555, p. 3; contains also the *Cantica Avicennae a magistro Armengando Blash de Montepesulano ex arabico in latinum translata, cum castigationibus clarissimi philosophi ac medici Andreae Bellunensis*). The non-naturals are enumerated and named as such in the above Latin version of Avicenna's *Cantica: aer, cibus et potus, somnus et vigilia, motus et quies, evacuatio et repletio, passiones animae* (ibid., p. 568). In O. C. Gruner's translation, *A Treatise on the Canon of Medicine of Avicenna*, London, 1930, the six are designated "causes" but not "non-naturals" (p. 30). Possibly the solution of the puzzle in nomenclature raised by the term "non-natural" lies in some confusion on the part of the Latin translators of "necessary factor" with "that which is neither" wholesome nor unwholesome. Galen's use of the phrases *kata physin* (*secundam naturam*) and *para physin* (*praeter naturam*) might have then suggested *non-naturales* as an intermediate term. Levinus Lemnius (1505–1568) can be taken as representative of another explanation of the term. Referring to the above passage in Galen's *Ars medica*, he states that Galen's conserving causes are termed non-naturals by later physicians not because they are praeternatural but because they are things external rather than within us, "... vocantur autem Galeno *causae conseruatrices, quod corporis nostri constitutionem conseruare idonea sunt, modo iis commodo atque opportune utamur* (*artium medicae* 85). Recentiores medici res non naturales vocant; non quod praeter naturam existant, sed quoniam extra nos constitutae sunt, nec nobis insitae ..." (*De habitu et constitutione corpore, quam Graeci krasin, triuiales complexionem vocant, Libri II ...* Frankfort, 1596, pp. 53–4. English translation by Thomas Newton, *The Touchstone of the Complexions*, London, 1581, p. 47).

72. (1) *ingesta*, (2) *retenta*, (3) *applicata externa corpori*, (4) *gesta*, including the *animi affectus* (*Institutiones medicae, digestae ab Hermanno Boerhaave, ed. Leydensis sexta, Lugduni Batavorum*, 1746, pp. 376–9).

73. Ibid., p. 379: "*Hoc nomine donatae, quia usu, vel abusu, bonae naturales, aut malae contranaturales, fieri queunt*".

74. Gaub, *Institutiones*, §522–6.

75. "*... cogitandi materies ...*".

76. "*Internos autem, quos vocant ...*".

77. Harry Austryn Wolfson, "The Internal Senses in Latin, Arabic and Hebrew Philosophic Texts", *Harvard Theological Review*, 28:69–133,

1935. Gaub sometimes confuses interior awareness of the Cartesian variety, i.e. the self-awareness of the *cogito*, with inner sense experience of the older kind. Descartes, in reflecting on the problem of pain from a phantom limb, finds the evidence of the interior senses just as uncertain as that of the exterior senses (Descartes, *Meditations touchant la première philosophie*, p. 322).

78. Maurice Merleau-Ponty, *The Phenomenology of Perception;* translated from the French by Colin Smith, London, 1962, pp. 75–89. His analysis of the evidence shows that the "phantom limb" can be adequately explained neither in purely physiological nor purely psychological terms. What fails in our explanations is a way of linking "third person" processes with personal acts.

79. "... *mores hominum* ...".

80. Robert Fuchs (*Puschmann's Handbuch der Geschichte der Medizin*), 3 vols., Leipzig, 1902–05, vol. 1, p. 235) calls the correspondence between Hippocrates and Democritus a product of the school of rhetoric at Kos under the first Roman emperors. See also Werner Jaeger, *Paideia: the Ideals of Greek Culture*, translated by Gilbert Highet, 3 vols., Oxford, 1944, vol. 3, p. 297, note 58a.

81. Littré's translation is *Tous les hommes doivent connaître l'art de médecine, ô Hippocrate ... Je pense que la connaissance de la philosophie est sœur de la médecine et vit sous le même toit; en effet, la philosophie délivre l'âme* (psychen) *des passions* (patheôn), *et la médecine enlève au corps les maladies. L'esprit* (noos) *croit, tant qu'est présente la santé, à laquelle il est bien que veille un homme sage; mais quand la constitution corporelle souffre, l'esprit n'a plus même de souci pour le soin de la vertu* (aretês) (Hippocrates/ Littré, vol. 9, p. 393–5). A different meaning is given to the Greek text in the Latin translation used by Gaub: *augescere mentem, cum adest sanitas, adeoque huic ut prospiciant, qui recte sentiunt, consentaneum esse; ubi vero corporis habitus dolet, nec mentem ad virtutis meditationem esse alacrem.*

82. See Note 5.

83. Galen/Kühn, vol. IV, pp. 767–8.

84. Ibid., pp. 810–11.

85. "... *mores temperamentum corporis sequi* ...".

86. Plato, *Timaeus* 86–8; *Charmides* 156d.

87. "*Hunc errorem quasi radicem malorum omnium stirpitus philosophia se extracturam pollicetur*" (Cicero, *Tusculan Disputations*, with an English translation by J. E. King, London, 1927, reprinted 1960, IV, xxxviii).

88. "... *at cum in corporis compagine haec inoleverint, vix ita eruere possunt, ut non usque et usque recurrant ... Radicem in corpore defixam evellere oportet* ...".

89. "... *tantus tamen vir non potuit unum Alcibiadem a furore removere, neque a ferocia sanare*". Hermann Boerhaave, *Praelectiones Academica*

de Morbis Nervorum, quas ex auditorum manuscriptis collectas edi curavit Jacobus van Eems, medicus Leydensis, Lugduni Batavorum, 1761, Tom. II, p. 394.

90. "... *in omni temperamento aliqua intemperies sit* ...".

91. "... *animi morbos* ...".

92. In the Hippocratic treatise, "On the Nature of Man", it is stated that the body is made up of blood, phlegm, yellow bile and black bile and that man enjoys health when the powers (*dynameis*), amounts and mixture are perfectly compounded (Hippocrates/Littré, vol. 6, pp. 39–41). Alcmeon, whose writings precede those of the Hippocratic corpus, holds that health is the equality of rights of the functions wet, dry, cold, hot, bitter, sweet, and the rest (Kathleen Freeman, *Ancilla to the Pre-Socratic Philosophers*, Oxford, 1952, p. 40).

93. Galen/Kühn, vol. I, *De temperamentis*, pp. 519, 559, 572–3.

94. Ibid., vol. XIX, pp. 485–96, *De humoribus*. This treatise is regarded as spurious by Robert Fuchs (Puschmann, vol. 1, p. 391), but this is of no importance for our purposes, since it was nonetheless a part of the Galenical tradition.

95. "... *Graeci* ... sôphrosynên *vocant, quam soleo equidem tum temperantiam, tum moderationem appellare.*" (*Tusculan Disputations*, III, viii).

96. Ibid., IV, xiii. This passage in Cicero resembles very much a passage in Galen (Galen/Kühn, vol. XIX, *Definitiones medicae*, Def. CXXX). Robert Fuchs attributes these definitions to Pneumaticists of the third century (p. 39). In both instances the virtues of the mind and body are named and an analogy drawn between temperance of the mind (*sôphrosynê*) and right constitution of the body (*krasis*).

97. *De humoribus*, cited in Note 94 above.

98. Gaub, *Institutiones*, §40.

99. Ludwig Edelstein, *The Hippocratic Oath* (Supplements to the *Bulletin of the History of Medicine*, No. 1), Baltimore, 1943, p. 23.

100. Plato, *Timaeus*, translated by R. G. Bury, London, 1952, pp. 86, 87.

101. A. E. Taylor, *A Commentary on Plato's Timaeus*, Oxford, 1928, pp. 619–20.

102. Galen/Kühn, vol. XIX, *Definitiones medicae*, Def. CIV.

103. The reader may be interested in hearing a modern voice on the temperaments. They are, writes Kretschmer, partly determined humorally, through the make-up of the blood. They are aspects of the *psyché*, correlated with bodily structure, and their bodily representative is the brain-endocrine apparatus (Ernst Kretschmer, *Körperbau und Character, 5te und 6te Auflage*, Berlin, 1926, p. 208). "Humorally" here simply means by way of substances, chiefly of endocrine gland origin, circulating in the fluids of the body. The "temperaments" have now become aspects of the *psyché*, with correlates in the body.

104. *"Venio nunc ad illa animi vitia, quae proprie morbis accenseri solent, quibusque si homo adfligitur, aegrotare eum dicimus."* "Morbus" in Gaub's time was applied to more or less specific bodily diseases, although it can be extended to cover various forms of mental disturbance. "Aegrotare" is to fall ill in body or mind.

105. *"... affectiones animi suo quodam jure ad aegritudines etiam referri debent ... mollius ea propter nomen passim accepere; ne omnes male sani diceremur. Et profecto ubi cuncti sunt Polyphemi, quis unoculum arguat?"* "Aegritudines" are illnesses involving the mind or body. Gaub makes use of the phrase "male sani" which occurs also in the *Tusculan Disputations*. Cicero compares bodily disease and emotional disturbances as follows: *"... ut aegrotatio in corpore, sic aegritudo in animo"* (*Tusculan Disputations* III, x).

106. *"... ex labefacttao corporis statu oriuntur ... Maniam volo, melancholiam, phrenitidem, desipientias febriles, furores uterinos, rabiem ex morsu animalium rabidorum natam, catalepsin, ceteros".*

107. Bartholomew Perdulcis, for example, quoting the sixth-century physician Aëtios, calls phrenitis an *"inflammationem membranarum cerebri, quae febrem acutam, et mentis perturbationem inducit"* (*De morbis animi*, Paris, 1639, p. 9).

108. *Amaltheum Castello-Brunonianum, sive Lexicon Medicum*, Patavii, 1746, p. 149.

109. Gaub's citation reads Th. Bartholinus' *Acta Medica Hafniensis*, vol. V, p. 162. The full citation is *Thomae Bartholini Acta Medica et Philosophica*, ann. 1677, 1678, 1679, 5 vols. in 4, Hafniae, 1680, vol. V, pp. 162–3. The boy was fourteen years old, and was said to have spoken Latin fluently during his last illness, where three days before he had been unable to decline a noun and an adjective properly.

110. See Note 63.

111. Schenck von Grafenberg, *Observationum medicarum rararum, novarum, admirabilium et monstrosarum volumen*, Frankfort, 1602, *Lib. IV*, p. 566.

112. *Gregor Horstii, Marcellus Donatus, editio nova, De medica historia mirabili*, Frankfort, 1664, Bk. IV, p. 298, *"... rotae atque ignis tormento perempta, ita a iustitiae iudicibus damnatum, quod blanditiis pueros alliciens inque domum introducens enecaret, et sale condiret".*

113. Ibid., p. 298, *"Hanc nos mulierem profecto pica morbo laborasse arbitramur, non enim ita crudelem existimandum ipsam fuisse".* For instances of beneficial compulsive appetites see Gaub II, 31, 34.

114. Ibid., p. 299, *"... mihi credite vbi experti essetis, quam palatum delectet humana caro, qui a liberorum esu abstinet inueniretur nemo."* Gaub cites the case from Donatus, who had it in turn from Hector Boethius' *History of the Scots*.

115. *"... cum hujus modi ... morbo obnoxia".*

116. See Note 72.

117. Gaub, *Institutiones*, §59.

118. "... *cum materie* ... *sine hac* ...".

119. Kühn, in Galen/Kühn, vol. I, LVII, "... *cum materia, aut sine illa* ...".

120. Ibid.

121. *Francisci Mercurii Helmontii, Observationes circa hominem et ejusque morbos*, p. 33. Not verified by me. See Gaub II, Note 227, and text.

122. Littré, vol. 9, p. 233: "*Iêtros gar philosophos isotheos*", translated as "*Le médecin philosophe est égal aux dieux*". Jones translates it as "for a physician who is a lover of wisdom is the equal of a god" (*Hippocrates, with an English translation by W. H. S. Jones*, Loeb Library, Cambridge, 1952, 4 vols., vol. 2, p. 287).

123. Gaub's citation reads *Th. Barthol., Act. Med. Hafniensis*, vol. V, p. 169. Full reference as in Note 109. Borrichius notes that loss of memory is a rare accompaniment of venesection, and describes a case in an elderly ecclesiastic. He remarks also that terror may abolish the memory.

124. Gaub's citation reads *Naudé, Considérations politiques*. The reference is to Gabriel Naudé's *Considérations politiques sur les coups d'état*, Paris, 1627.

125. Bartholomaeus Perdulcis, loc. cit., p. 50.

126. Galen/Daremberg, pp. 56, 57.

127. Margaret A. Murray, *The Witch Cult in Modern Europe*, London, 1921, reprinted 1962, app. V (flying ointments) by A. J. Clark, pp. 279–80.

Notes

Essay of 1763

1. "*Doleo equidem vehementer, Mimum, an Momum? Gallulum ...* *putidum automatis sui humani scilicet! partum edidisse ...*".

2. Aram Vartanian, *La Mettrie's* L'Homme Machine, *A Study in the Origins of an Idea*, Princeton, 1960, p. 1.

3. Raymond Savioz, *Mémoires autobiographiques de Charles Bonnet de Genève*, (Diss.), Paris, 1948, p. 193. The quotation given here comes from a letter written by Gaub to Bonnet dated 25 March, 1761. Gaub adds, with reference to Bonnet's *Essai Analytique*, that in "seeing you push the mechanism of the faculties of the mind to the ultimate degree it becomes clear that thought cannot be deduced as a true effect, and that one absolutely must have recourse to an active principle of entirely different nature, which winds the machine and is the source of what is properly called thought".

4. Ibid., p. 193.

5. Vartanian, p. 152; Gaub I, §50.

6. Vartanian, p. 153; Gaub I, §30.

7. Vartanian, p. 173; Gaub I, §85.

8. Vartanian, p. 173; Gaub I, §86.

9. Vartanian, p. 173; Gaub I, §86.

10. Vartanian, p. 173; Gaub I, §86.

11. Vartanian, p. 155; Gaub I, §60.

12. Vartanian, p. 207.

13. Boerhaave, *Institutiones*, 1746, p. 9.

14. Ibid., p. 10.

15. Ibid., p. 10.

16. Ibid., pp. 361–2.

17. Hermann Boerhaave, *Opera omnia medica, oratio II, de usu ratiocinii mechanici in medicina habita in auditorio magno 24 Septembris, a. 1702*, Venice, 1747.

18. Ibid., p. 448.

19. Ibid., p. 449.

20. Ibid., p. 451.

21. Ibid., p. 456.

22. An interesting definition of "machina" given by Asconius in the first century A.D. runs, *inventum, in quo, non tam materiae ratio ducitur, quam manus, atque artus* (Forcellini, *Totius latinitatis lexicon*, 3rd ed., Schneeberg, 1833, 4 vols., vol. 3, p. 2). In other words, it is matter arranged in accordance with the plan of an inventor, by art rather than by nature.

23. Robert Boyle, "A Free Inquiry into the Vulgarly Received Notion of Nature", *Works*, London, 1772, vol. 5, p. 211.

24. Augustin Fasch, *Disputatio inauguralis medica de* autocheiria *praeside Dn. Augustino Henrico Faschio . . . subjicit Fredericus Hoffmanus, Jenae*, 31 Jan. 1681, p. 3.

25. Descartes, *Les Passions de l'Âme*, p. 697. The comparison antedates Descartes. Luis Vives (1492–1540) used it, as Robert Burton points out, "For our body is like a clock; if one wheel be amiss, all the rest are disordered . . . as Lodovicus Vives, in his *Fable of Man*, hath elegantly declared" (Burton, *Anatomy of Melancholy*, Pt. 1, Sec. 1, Mem. 3, Subs. 2, p. 109).

26. Ibid., p. 696. Elsewhere Descartes states that "*. . . moi, venant à prendre garde que le principe par lequel nous sommes nourris est entièrement distingué de celui par lequel nous pensons, j'ai dit que le nom d'*âme *. . . doit être seulement entendu de ce principe par lequel nous pensons*" (Descartes, *Réponses de l'auteur aux cinquième objections faites par Monsieur Gassendi*, p. 482).

27. Gottfried W. Leibniz, in Georg Ernst Stahl, *Negotium otiosum seu skiamachia*, Halle, 1720, *Dubia sive . . . animadversiones, circa assertiones aliquas Theoriae Medicae Verae*, p. 1, "*. . . Hinc consequens est, omnem rerum affectionem, omnem in rebus eventum ex ipsarum Natura statuque posse derivari; & speciatim, quicquid in Materia evenit, ex praecedenti materiae Statu, per leges mutationum oriri. Atque hoc est, quod volunt aut velle debent, qui dicunt, omnia in corporibus Mechanice explicari posse.*" This is precisely the formulation used by Bertrand Russell in a recent discussion in which he takes Gilbert Ryle to task for seeming to think that because physicists have abandoned billiard ball mechanism they have abandoned mechanism altogether. The question is, says Russell, do the equations of physics combined with data as to the distribution of energy at some given time suffice to determine what has happened or what will happen to portions of matter not below a certain minimum size? Could an ideal physicist, in other words, calculate what anyone would say throughout the rest of his life, since speaking involves the movement of matter? (Bertrand Russell, "What is Mind?", *Journal of Philosophy*, 55: 5, 1958.

28. "*. . . nullum tamen a machinis illis sola illarum dispositione edi posse in humano corpore motum absque animae concursu*" (Joseph Carrère, *Dissertatio medica de vitali corporis et animae foedere*, Perpignan, 1758, pp. 51–2).

29. W. Smith, M.D., *A Dissertation on the Nerves*. London, 1768, pp. 16–17. This work has been called an unacknowledged paraphrase of a plagiarism by Nicholas Robinson of a sermon by Andrew Snape (Richard Hunter and Ida Macalpine, *Three Hundred Years of Psychiatry*, London, 1963, p. 303).

30. The effects of Descartes's doctrine among some of his disciples were described by Fontaine: "They thought nothing of dissecting animals alive in order to study the circulation, and mocked those who claimed that the beasts felt pain like themselves ... they said that they were clocks and that the cries were no more than the noise of a little spring that had been moved", cited by Fernand Louis-Mueller in *Histoire de la psychologie de l'antiquité à nos jours*, Paris, 1960, p. 209. It was unusual but not entirely without precedent for Descartes to deny feelings to animals. Galen states that there are those *qui vel nullum animal brutum concupiscere aut irasci ... affirmarent* (*Claudii Galeni, De placitis Hippocratis et Platonis ... recensuit et explanavit Iwanus Mueller*, Leipzig, 1874, vol. I, pp. 168–9).

31. Johann Pauli, *Disputatio medica inauguralis de animi commotionum vi medica ... praeside Dn. Johanne Wilhelmo Pauli ... submittit Christianus Mentz, 30 April 1700, Lipsiae*. Pauli (1658–1723) held several chairs, including those of anatomy, surgery and pathology, at Leipzig.

32. "... *animum in duas partes diviserunt, alteram rationis participem, alteram expertem: in participe rationis posuere* [Cicero: *ponunt*] *tranquillitatem, id est, placidam quietamque constantiam, in illa altera motus turbidos tum irae, tum cupiditatis, contrarios inimicosque rationi.*" (*Tusculan Disputations*, IV, v).

33. Descartes, *Les Passions de l'Âme*, pp. 718, 719. The Cartesian explanation is well within the tradition of Christian dualism here: "For the flesh lusteth against the Spirit, and the Spirit against the flesh: and these are contrary the one to the other: so that ye cannot do the things that ye would" (Galatians 5, 17).

34. Cited by Rudolf Eisler, *Wörterbuch der Philosophischen Begriffe, 2te Aufl.*, Berlin, 1904, 2 vols., vol. 2, p. 324. *Anima secundum sui officium variis nuncupatur nominibus. Dicitur namque anima dum vegetat, spiritus dum contemplantur, sensus dum sensit, animus dum sapit: dum intelligit, mens: dum discernit, ratio: dum recordatur, memoria: dum vult, voluntas. Ista tamen non differunt in substantia quemadmodum differunt in nominibus: quoniam omnia ista una anima est, proprietates quidem diversae* (*De spir. et an.*, 13).

35. Other writers make similar comments. Laehr, for example, lists a seventeenth-century work by Rorarius entitled *Quod animalia bruta saepe ratione utantur melius homine* (Heinrich Laehr, *Die Literatur der Psychiatrie, Neurologie und Psychologie im XVIII. Jahrhundert*, Berlin, 1895, p. 29).

36. "... *ferreae naturae* ...".

37. Pliny Secundus, according to Gellius, reported that hellebore could be taken with greatest safety on the *island* of Anticyra but the location of this island is unknown (*The Attic Nights of Aulus Gellius, with an English translation by John C. Rolfe*, London, 1927 (Loeb Library), revised and reprinted 1961, 3 vols., vol. 3, XVII, xv).

38. Gerard van Swieten, *Commentaria in Hermanni Boerhaavii Aphorismos*, Hildburghausen, 1754, vol. III, p. 334. Gaub apparently meant to add an additional pun of his own, since he wrote "... *quod inter Italos extare perhibent* ...".

39. M. (Simon-André) Tissot, *Essai sur les maladies des gens du monde*, 2nd ed., Lausanne, 1770.

40. Ibid., p. IX. He adds that a book on medicine of the court has been written by the physician of the King of Denmark, but as it is in German he has been unable to read it.

41. Ibid., pp. 24, 30, 52. Tissot considers the non-naturals, the *choses non-naturelles*, systematically.

42. Ibid., pp. 57, 58.

43. Ibid., pp. 61–2.

44. Ibid., p. 63.

45. Ibid., pp. 35–43. Tissot states that, in general, strong emotions have more influence on the health of the body than the quality of the food, or even of the air.

46. Gaub, *Institutiones*, §18.

47. "... *mentem perturbatam* ...".

48. "... *recta ratio* ...".

49. *Tusculan Disputations*, IV, xviii. Cicero uses this argument to reject the Peripatetic doctrine of the "limit" (within which strong emotions were to be held to a beneficial mean) in favor of the Stoic doctrine of the desirability of the complete suppression of emotions (*apatheia*). The Peripatetic position, in other words, was that even strong emotions were beneficial if properly managed. Seneca uses Cicero's illustration and argument in his essay on anger (*De ira*, I, vii, 2–4). Gaub rejects the Stoic position in II, §48. It is, of course, incompatible with the doctrine of the non-naturals.

50. Descartes, *Les Passions de l'Âme*, art, 41, p. 715.

51. "... *quae mens suopte impetu conturbata patrat, cum cogitatione in bonum malumve, quod rebus subesse credit* ...". See Gaub I, 34 and commentary.

52. Cicero says that the countenance is dominated by the eyes and is the image of the mind; the face is the one part of the body that has as many significant changes as there are emotions (*Cicero, De oratore, with an English translation by H. Rackham*, London, 1942 (Loeb Library), reprinted 1960, 2 vols., vol. 2, III, lix). Seneca, whose description of the outward appearance of an angry man all of our authors seem to have read, states that every violent emotion affects the face in one way or another, and anger most of all (*Seneca, Moral Essays, with an English translation by John W. Basore*, London, 1928 (Loeb Library) reprinted 1958, 3 vols., vol. 1, *De ira*, I, 1). Basing his stand on the Stoic belief that reality is corporeality Seneca argues that the emotions are corporeal, anger, love, sorrow and the rest, since they actively change our outward

appearance and whatever acts is corporeal, *quod facit, corpus est.* If emotions are corporeal, so are diseases of the mind, *morbi animorum* (*Seneca, ad Lucilium epistulae morales, with an English translation by Richard M. Gummere*, London, 1925 (Loeb Library) reprinted 1953, 3 vols., vol. 3, "On the Corporeality of Virtue", Epist. CVI). In giving the reasons why the medical school of Empiricists rejected the vivisection of men in the investigation of disease, Celsus writes that the body undergoes external change in the face of fear and pain, hence it is likely that the softer internal parts are even more severely affected (Celsus, *De medicina, Prooemium,* 41).

53. Descartes, *Les Passions de l'Âme,* arts. 112–13, p. 747.

54. Gaub, *Institutiones,* §542.

55. See Gaub I, §38–42.

56. Gaub's words, *neque enim brevi semper furore ira detonat,* echo those of Horace, *ira furore brevis est,* anger is a brief madness. Galen, too, finds that the behavior of angry men toward their slaves is like that of the insane. They kick, strike and beat them (Galen/Kühn, vol. V, *De propriarum animi cuiusque affectuum dignotione et curatione,* pp. 1–57).

57. . . . *nisi prudens gratiosae facultatis judicium intercesserit.*

58. Hermann Boerhaave, *Praelectiones de morbis nervorum, quas ex auditorum manuscriptis collectas edi curavit Jacobus van Eems, medicus Leydensis,* Leiden, 1761, 2 vols., vol. 1, pp. 478–9. Boerhaave (1668–1738) taught physiology, pathology, surgery, pharmacology, chemistry and botany at the University of Leiden.

59. J. N. Pechlin, *Observationum physico-medicarum libri tres,* Hamburg, 1691, Obs. XIX, p. 440. Pechlin (1644–1706) was professor of medicine in Kiel.

60. Ibid., Obs. XXV, p. 445.

61. J. F. Zückert, *Von den Leidenschaften, 2te Aufl.,* Berlin, 1768, pp. 50–5. Zückert (1737–1778), a physician, gave up the practice of medicine because of poor health, and devoted himself to writing.

62. Corp, *An Essay on the Changes Produced in the Body by the Operations of the Mind, by the late Doctor Corp of Bath,* London, 1791, pp. 55–9.

63. Raimund Laroque, "De l'influence des passions sur l'économie animale, considérée dans les quatre âges de la vie". *Collections des thèses soutenues a l'école de Montpellier en l'an V et l'an VI, Montpellier, l'an VI,* p. 12.

64. Morgagni, *The Seats and Causes of Diseases investigated by anatomy . . . translated from the Latin of John Baptist Morgagni . . . by Benjamin Alexander, M.D.,* 3 vols., London, 1769, facsimile ed., New York, 1960, vol. 2, pp. 212–13. Morgagni (1682–1771) was professor of medicine at Padua from 1712 to the time of his death. The above work was first published in 1761. On page 213 Morgagni cites the case of a patient described in the *Medicina rationalis systematica* of Friedrich H. Hoffmann. The febrile paroxysms and intermittent

attacks of jaundice of this patient are said to be the consequence of a "preceding commotion of mind". Friedrich Theodor Frerichs, a well-known German clinician of the mid-nineteenth century, makes use of Morgagni's explanation in his own discussion of emotional jaundice. Physicians, Frerichs writes, have at all times maintained that jaundice can be produced by functional derangements of the nervous system, possibly as the result of a spasm of the bile ducts or small bowel obstructing the passage of bile, but he finds that jaundice of this kind develops much more rapidly after the onset of the emotion than after complete closure of the bile duct. He suggests that a derangement of nervous function leads to an accumulation of bile in the blood by interrupting the circulation of blood through the liver. The interruption in turn might be due to narrowing of the blood-vessels of the liver. In the violent emotions of anger and fright, the epigastrium is suddenly compressed. This is followed by difficulty in breathing, a feeling of suffocation and at times vomiting. The skin becomes pale and soon after takes on a yellow color. Meanwhile, large quantities of pale urine are excreted. The limited loss of coloring matter in the urine, Frerichs believes, influences the rapid appearance of jaundice of the skin. In such cases the yellow color appears within a few hours, sometimes within an even shorter space of time. Frerichs cites an instance described by Villermé. Two young men drew their swords in the course of a quarrel, whereupon one of them suddenly turned yellow. The other dropped his weapon, terrified in turn by this sudden change of color. Frerichs says that while one may be inclined to doubt such stories there are numerous observations indicating that under circumstances of emotional upset jaundice can develop more rapidly than after ligation of the common bile duct. One must be careful in coming to a decision about these stories, he adds, since there are countries in which the popular belief that jaundice depends on the emotions is so widespread that almost every case is attributed to this cause. He notes that emotional jaundice usually passes off without further consequences, although exceptional cases occur in which death ensues after a few days amid delirium, convulsions and other severe nervous symptoms (Friedrich Theodor Frerichs, *Klinik der Leberkrankheiten*, Braunschweig, 1858, 2 vols., vol. I, pp. 165–7).

65. Morgagni, pp. 213–14.
66. Gaub, *Institutiones*, §633–49.
67. Ibid., §542.
68. Johanne Baptista Scaramucci, *De hydrophobo ex irae impetu tali, Acta Eruditorum, N. IV, Lipsiae,* April 1702, p. 147.
69. Ibid., "... *ut venemum ejusmodi rabiosum constituere facile psssint, quod communicantur postmodum, mediante morsu*".
70. Boerhaave/van Eems, p. 483. Boerhaave calls it the *vis sensorii communis*.

71. Ibid., pp. 555–6.

72. Corp, pp. 57–8.

73. Job 32, 2, 3, 6, 19: "Then kindled the wrath of Elihu . . . against Job . . . . I am young and ye are very old; wherefore I was afraid . . . . Behold, my belly is as wine which hath no vent; it is ready to burst like new bottles."

74. Georg Stahl, *Ueber den mannigfaltigen Einfluss von Gemüthsbewegungen auf den menschlichen Körper*, translated by Bernward J. Gottlieb (*Sudhoff's Klassiker der Medizin*), Leipzig, 1961. William Harvey (1578–1657) describes a similar case. He knew a prudent man, he tells us, who was angered by an affront afflicted on him by a more powerful person. Revenge was out of the question. He tried to swallow his hatred but it mounted daily and he succumbed at last to a strange disease characterized by oppression and pain in the region of the heart. At autopsy the heart was found to be enormously enlarged. Harvey's comment—"so great is the power of confined or enclosed blood, so dynamic is it"—shows the extent to which he was influenced by older ideas regarding the circulation of the blood even after having promulgated his own (*William Harvey, The Circulation of the Blood and Other Writings, translated by Kenneth J. Franklin*, London, 1963, "A Second Essay to Jean Riolan", p. 163).

75. ". . . *atrabilaria humorum spissitas, acrimonia . . .*".

76. Gaub, *Institutiones*, §282, 285, 304. Diarrhea and jaundice are further effects of grief (Ibid., §542).

77. The condition referred to here, now known as hypersomnia or pathologically excessive sleep, occasionally follows brain injury and may also be of psychogenic origin, as Gaub believed.

78. Montaigne, p. 32–3.

79. Zückert, pp. 47–50.

80. Corp, p. 86–7.

81. Smith, p. 176.

82. According to Stahl sorrow most frequently causes chronic disease. He mentions one case (not his own) of a woman who fell dead on hearing of the unexpected death of her son (Stahl/Gottlieb, p. 33). Descartes, in discussing an ailment of his illustrious correspondent, the Princess Elisabeth, recalls the troubles of her house (her father had lost the throne of Bohemia in 1620) and states that sorrow is the most common cause of a lingering fever (Descartes, *Lettre à Elisabeth, 18 mai, 1645*, p. 1182). Here as elsewhere when dealing with the emotions and bodily health Descartes forgets his own theory (which makes the *felt* emotion a result rather than a cause of physiological processes in the body, since the felt emotion is nothing more than the mind's awareness of these processes) and reverts to the traditional view. Again, he tells her that someone with no real cause for complaint can fall victim to a dangerous cough as a result of altering his circulation and breathing by

busying the mind with sorrowful thoughts, in fact, his own mother had died a few days after his birth due to a disease induced by displeasure (ibid., p. 1188). Descartes also described, in his own terminology, the conditional reflex of modern physiology (the substitution of one stimulus for another as the trigger releasing a pattern of behavior) and made use of it to account for the various ways in which the emotions are expressed. The union of mind and body is so close, he writes, that once a certain bodily action has been linked with a certain thought, the appearance of either one will cause the other to manifest itself as well (*Les Passions de l'Âme*, art. 107, pp. 744–5). Sorrow caused some people to lose their appetites and others to overeat (Descartes remarked that he belonged in the second class), because in the one case sorrow was initially associated with harmful food and in the other case with lack of food— sorrow and aversion for food becoming associated thereafter in the first case and sorrow and desire for food in the second (*Lettre à Elisabeth, 5 mai, 1646*, p. 1231). Various writers comment on the effects of sorrow in animals: Agrippa attributes to an excess of sorrow the death of dogs after the death of their masters (Henry Cornelius Agrippa von Nettesheim, *De occulta philosophia . . . Lugduni, per Beringos fratres*, n.d., vol. 1, p. 101) and Gellius, another of Gaub's sources, tells the story of an amorous dolphin who died of grief after the loss of his beloved, a young boy. They were buried in the same tomb, says Gellius (*Attic Nights*, VI, viii).

83. Gaub, *Institutiones*, §542. Galen says that envy, the state in which the pleasure of one person is disagreeable to another, is the most painful of the emotions (Galen/Kühn, vol. V, *De proprium animi cuiusque affectuum dignotione et curatione*, cap. vii).

84. Gaub names "*dolores, angores, aphonias, lipothymias, tetanos, tremores, convulsiones, epilepsias, catalepses, apoplexias, paralyses, deliria multifaria, mortes subitaneas*". For "catalepses" see commentary to §81 of the first lecture.

85. Gaub, *Institutiones*, §542.

86. Stahl/Gottlieb, pp. 33, 34.

87. *timor.*

88. called here *terror* or *metus.*

89. Philip Holland, *Dissertatio medica inauguralis, pauca de mente in corpus effectibus, exponens . . . ex auctoritate D. Gulielmi Robertson . . . subjicit Phillipus Holland*, Edinburgh, 1782, p. 33.

90. Zückert, p. 43.

91. Corp, p. 84.

92. Ibid., pp. 66–68.

93. Ibid., p. 71.

94. Ibid., pp. 68–69.

95. Johann Juncker, *Dissertatio inauguralis medica de noxa atque utilitate animi pathematum seu adfectuum in medicina, praeside Dn. Joanne Junckero, auctor Ionness Godofriedus Grunou*, Berlin, 1745, p. 19.

Juncker (1697–1759), professor of medicine of Halle, was a follower of Stahl.

96. Valangin, loc. cit., p. 333.

97. Ibid., pp. 335–6.

98. Pechlin, Obs. XXI, pp. 445–7.

99. Ibid., Obs. XXI, p. 444.

100. Ibid., Obs. XXIII, p. 449.

101. Ibid., Obs. XX, p. 443.

102. Ibid., Obs. XVIII, p. 437.

103. Holland, loc. cit., p. 33.

104. Corp, p. 72.

105. Smith, p. 165.

106. Graemius Mercer, *Dissertatio physico-medica inauguralis de pathematibus animi eorumque in corpus humanum effectibus . . . ex auctoritate D. Gulielmi Robertson . . . subjicit Graemius Mercer*, Edinburgh, 1784, pp. 35–6.

107. Valangin, p. 332.

108. Boerhaave/van Eems, p. 480.

109. Mercer, p. 35.

110. Holland, p. 32.

111. Ibid., p. 32.

112. Laroque, p. 13.

113. "*. . . animi intemperantia*", that is, an absence of *sôphrosynê*.

114. "*. . . fervens concitatusque animus suopte motu in venas medullasque diffuso patrat.*"

115. "*. . . hic fervor concitatioque animi inveteraverit et tamquam in venis medullisque insederit . . .*" (*Tusculan Disputations*, IV, x).

116. "*. . . atra bile, chlorosi, erotomania . . .*".

117. Dorland, *American Illustrated Medical Dictionary*, Philadelphia, 1951.

118. *Amaltheum Lexicon*, p. 334.

119. *Plutarch's Lives, with an English translation by Bernardotte Perrin* (Loeb Library), 11 vols., vol. IX, Demetrius XXXVIII, pp. 93–4. Pliny, however, ascribes the diagnosis to Kleombrotus, identified by Robert Fuchs as the father of Erasistratus (Puschmann, I, 297).

120. Of the extent to which the *sôma* could be affected by the *psychês pathê* (Galen/Kühn, vol. XIV, pp. 631–4). In his extended discussion of love-melancholy Burton mentions Galen's case among others, including those of Charicles, son of Polycles, whose ailment was diagnosed by Panacius, the love of Poliarchus and Argenis, etc. Valesius, according to Burton, denies the existence of a *pulsus amatorius*, but Avicenna confirms Galen on this point out of his own experience (*Anatomy of Melancholy*, Pt. 3, Sec. 2, Mem. 3). One of Burton's sources, Joseph Struth (1510–1568) a famous physician in his day, wrote a treatise on the pulse in which the effects of the emotions are described in great detail. Anger (*altum, magnum celerem, crebrum, vehementum*), joy

(*magnum, tardum, rarum, moderatum*), sorrow (*parvum, tardum, rarum, languidum*), and fear (*recens, celerem, inordinatum, inaequalem*) produce characteristic changes in the pulse. Struth agrees with Galen (he was one of Galen's Latin translators) that there is no proper pulse for love; it depends on the particular emotion aroused by circumstances (*Ars sphygmica seu pulsuum doctrina . . . a Josepho Struthio . . . Libris V*, Basel, 1602, Bk. IV, Cap. XIII, p. 219). Struth tells how he found out the name of the lover of a certain nobleman's wife by palpating her pulse as he casually mentioned the names of various acquaintances. One name, he writes, and that only, on repeated test caused her pulse to become *celerior, crebrior et languidor* (ibid., pp. 218–19). The emotions, Struth remarks, have the power to bring about amazing changes in the body (ibid., p. 214).

121. Juncker, p. 15.
122. Laroque, p. 10.
123. Valangin, p. 23.
124. Holland, p. 30.
125. Zückert, pp. 61–4. He mentions in passing that an outstanding description of "heartbreak" may be found in Richardson's *Clarissa*. A modern novelist's treatment of the subject, called to my attention by Henri Ellenberger, is of particular interest because the physician in the novel, Ellenberger believes, represents Charcot. The physician in the novel says of his patient that she is dying of love but we call it neurasthenia in order not to appear ignorant—"*Nous disons de neurasthénie parce que nous avons peur de sembler simples et ignorants si nous disons: d'amour*" (Marcel Prévost, *L'automne d'une femme*, Vienna, (n.d.)).
126. The Parisian physician Bartholomy Pardoux (1545–1611) treats of the pathology of love in some detail in his work on diseases of the mind, and although he is too early to be regarded as a contemporary of Gaub, his views are of interest in showing the doctrine of the non-naturals in action. He distinguishes uterine furors (nymphomania) from insane love, describing the former as an inordinate desire for sexual intercourse so unrestrained and wanton that the brain is affected and the sufferer driven mad. It begins as a difficulty (*in genere actionis laesae*) involving the natural and vital functions, as indicated by the immoderate desire coupled with depravity of the imagination and mind. The anatomical parts chiefly affected are the neck and mouth of the uterus. An ardor, an itch, an insatiable appetite, is communicated from here via the diaphragm to the brain. The external causes of the disease are a hot climate, the season of summer, an excess of spicy and aromatic foods (including onions and artichokes), unmixed wine, soft beds, an indolent and leisurely life, and lascivious talk, shows and books. The internal causes are a hot, moist temperament and a bilious constitution. The latter is associated with an abundance of serous, salty, biting humor that

stimulates the sexual parts and (aided by retention and putrefaction of the generative seed) rises through the spinal medulla and the nerves to affect the brain with "foul vapors" and disturb the chief faculty of the mind (*Bartholomaeus Perdulcis, De morbis animi,* Paris, 1639, pp. 49–53). The treatment offered follows Galenical lines. Since hot and moist qualities are predominant the diet should be refrigerating (*contraria contrariis sanantur*). Appropriate foods to produce this effect include cucumbers, prunes, apples cooked together with the peripheral parts of animals, chicken soup, lettuce, chicory, and purslain. Cold water, beer and barley-water are suitable for drinking. Cold baths, a narrow bed provided with a wool mattress and light coverings, and fitting employment to keep the patient always busy complete this part of the treatment. If the maiden is nubile she should (in accordance with the advice of Hippocrates) be given an honest and lawful husband, for no other remedy is so effective against this disease. If this cannot be done she should be distracted by pious reading and decent conversation. Suitable exhortations are to be employed, such as the rewards of virtue to be expected if she recovers and the opprobium to be looked for if she does not, e.g. she may be told that the virgins of Miletus affected by this disease were driven naked through the market place. Secondly, evacuants are to be used, such as frequently applied clysters of milk and decoctions of lettuce, plums, apples, helxines, violets and water-lilies. Blood may be withdrawn from both arms followed by strong purgation and warm baths. The saphenous veins may be tapped in the region of the ankles in order to provoke the menses. Cupping after scarification of the thighs and the application of leeches to the fundament in order to promote hemorrhoids complete this aspect of the treatment. Thirdly, local applications to the uterus are employed: decoctions of *agnus castus* (the chaste willow) and pessaries impregnated with the juices of coriander, rue and purslain (ibid., pp. 50, 51). Pardoux deals with love-sickness, *amor insanus,* in a separate chapter of his book. It is more commonly seen in men, he says, since they are of a warmer temperament than women. He defines the disease as a kind of melancholy affect or emotion due to an intemperance of the body which has been transmitted to the mind. If long persistent *amor insanus* dries out the brain and gives rise to delirium. The cause is a corruption of love, aroused by the sight of an attractive person of the opposite sex, and the afflicted individuals display a mixture of joy, sorrow, hope, fear and anxiety. The sensual and animal appetites and the concupiscible power seated in the liver are aroused. The increased vital heat thus occasioned disturbs the reason, which then becomes the slave of desire as the imagination bends toward the loved object alone and rejects all else; this object becomes so fixed in the mind that all other concerns are neglected. All of the natural powers are occupied with the thought of the loved one. Hence the food in the stomach and the blood in the liver are faultily concocted, with the result that an insufficient quantity of crude partly "adust" blood enters the veins and is distributed throughout the body. According to Paul of Aegina, says Pardoux, the pulse is not remarkable in love-sickness unless a conflict arises in the mind. If sight or sound suddenly introduces the loved one into the mind of the sufferer his pulse at once loses all regularity. (Pardoux mentions Galen's case at this point.) Not only does the pulse vary, but the face is suffused with blood, the eyes are exhilarated, and the breathing is interrupted by sighs. If the disease is not appropriately treated the sufferer wastes away or falls into a mania and finally dies. It should be cured in the beginning by one of two modes of treatment: possession of the loved one, or the use of the medical art. The first is the most immediately effective course, but if it is not feasible we must turn to the second. An attempt to busy the mind with other cares is to be made, and the patient if pious should be warned that not only honor but eternal felicity may be lost by yielding to the desire. If this procedure fails seclusion, hunger, thirst and blows may be tried. The faults and vices of the loved one are to be pointed out and at the same time someone more beautiful, accomplished and superior is described— a new love often explodes an old. Love has no more ready tinder than idleness, therefore the patient should be kept constantly busy and diverted by spectacles, games, conversation, hunting, walking, and the exercise of arms—Pallas, Diana and Vesta do not succumb to Venus (Pardoux heavily adds that Pallas signifies war, Diana hunting, and Vesta frugality). Travel is to be recommended. If all of these measures fail, the disease should be treated with medicines, *more melancholicorum*, in the fashion of a melancholy, using enemas, blood-letting and decoctions of refrigerating and drying substances. Wine is forbidden, lawful sexual intercourse permitted, and quieting potions and frequent mild baths are recommended (ibid., pp. 51, 53). Cicero's discussion of the subject in the *Tusculan Disputations* is probably a source for some of the measures described here; the remainder are more or less Galenical. Of all emotions, according to Cicero, there is none more violent than love, *omnibus enim ex animi perturbationis est profecto nulla vehementior*. Love is a madness, *furor amoris*. Cicero recommends the substitution of other interests, cares and occupations. Travel and attempts to convince the victim that the object of the desire is of no importance or that the desire can easily be satisfied elsewhere are also helpful. Some think the old love can be driven out by a new, as one nail drives out another, *tamquam clavo clavum eiiciendum* (*Tusculan Disputations*, IV, xxxv).

127. See Notes II, 78. Montaigne writes that the Pope manifested "*tel exces de joye que la fièvre l'en print et en mourut*" (loc. cit., p. 34).
128. Valangin, p. 324.
129. Corp, p. 52.

130. Juncker, p. 12.

131. Boerhaave/van Eems, p. 533.

132. Polycrita of Naxos, Philippides, Diogaras of Rhodes and, best known of all, the Roman matron who was first overwhelmed with grief by the false report of her son's death at Cannae and later fell dead with joy when he returned alive (*Attic Nights*, Bk. III, xv). The story is repeated by Montaigne (loc. cit., p. 34). Joseph Struth offers a first-hand account of a Polish woman who was so overcome with joy over the honors showered on her son that she was "deprived of her powers and died a few days later" (*Ars sphygmica*, pp 215–16). He attributes the death to excessive joy (*laetitia*). Galen attributes death from an excess of joy to a dissolution or extreme relaxation of bodily strength, and he contrasts it with death from terror, which is due to a sudden diminution of vital heat (Galen/Kühn, vol. VII, *De symptomatum causis, lib.* ii, p. 193). All of these authorities and more are recited by Rabelais in one breath: "Just so the heart with excessive joy is inwardly dilated and suffereth a manifest resolution of the vital spirits, which may go so farre on, that it may thereby be deprived of nourishment, and by consequence of life itself. By this Pericharie or extremity of gladness as Galen saith, lib. 12 *method*, lib. 5 *de locis affectis*, and lib. 2 *de symptomatum causis*. And as it hath come to pass in former times witnesse Marcius Tullius, lib. 1, *quaest. Tuscul.*, Verrius, Aristotle, Titus Livius in his relation of the battel of Cannae, Plinius, lib. 7, cap. 32 and 34. A. Gellius lib. 3, c. 15 and many other writers, of Diagoras the Rhodian, Chilon, Sophocles, Dionysius the tyrant of Sicilie, Phillipides, Philemon, Polycrates, Philistion, M. Juventi, and others who died of joy, and as Avicen speaketh, in 2 canon et lib. *de viribus cordis*, of the Saffron, that it doth so rejoice the heart that, if you take of it excessively, it will by a superfluous resolution and dilatation deprive it altogether of life" *Works of Mr. Francis Rabelais* (reprint of Urquhart-Motteux translation), New York, 1932, 2 vols., vol. 1, p. 23).

133. ... *animus decerptus ex mente divina* ... *Tuscular Disputations*, V, xiii

134. It is an old clinical observation that one disease may cure or ameliorate another. Wagner von Jauregg's observation that remissions of syphilitic paresis sometimes followed intercurrent acute infections led him to introduce malaria therapy in the treatment of late syphilis of the central nervous system (Julius Wagner von Jauregg, "Die progressive paralyse", *Neue Deutsche Klinik*, Berlin, 1932, vol. 9, p. 161).

135. "... *gulosis, ebriosis, lustronibus, ceterisque intemperantiae asseclis* ...".

136. "... *a tota mente et a recta ratione defectio* ..." (*Tusculan Disputations*, IV, ix). See also Gaub I, §74, including commentary and Notes. There he uses the term *intemperies* for intemperance of the body.

137. Ibid., IV, x.

138. Ibid., IV, xii.

139. See Notes I, 95.
140. Galen/Kühn, vol. V, *De propriorum animi cuiusque affectuum digno-tione et curatione*, cap. vi.
141. Ibid., vol XIX, *Definitiones medicae*, Def. CXXX.
142. *Tusculan Disputations*, IV, xiii.
143. Scott Buchanan finds the essence of medical theory and practice in this dialogue (*The Doctrine of Signatures, A Defence of Theory in Medicine*, London, 1938). Leibbrand and Wettley regard it as astounding that modern proponents of psychosomatic medicine do not place this passage from the *Charmides* at the head of their literary endeavors (Werner Leibbrand and Annemarie Wettley, *Der Wahnsinn: Geschichte der abendländischen Psychopathologie*, Freiburg/München, 1961, p. 66). The passage does, in fact, appear as an epigraph in *Psychogenese und Psychotherapie körperlicher Symptome*, ed. by Oswald Schwarz, Wien, 1925. Pedro Lain-Entralgo, commenting on this epigraph in his study of the curative power of the word in classical antiquity, finds that a full understanding of Plato's rationalization of the curative word—especially of the *epôdê* into the *logos kalos*—requires a study of the *Phaedrus, Phaedo, Symposium, Republic* and *Laws*, in addition to the *Charmides*. He himself has accomplished the task in a thoroughly satisfying way in his book *La Curación por la Palabra en la Antigüedad Clásica*, Madrid, 1958, pp. 163–97.
144. *Charmides*, 156–7. Lamb's translation (Loeb Classical Library, London, 1955, p. 21) reads "certain doctors who attempt to practice the one method without the other", where Jowett's reads "attempt to be physicians of health and temperance separately" (Plato, *The Collected Dialogues*, New York, 1963, p. 103). Plato's backing helped give this idea a permanent place in medical thought. Among the many writers who cite the *Charmides* we find Burton—"... for, as the body works upon the mind, by his bad humours, ... so, on the other side, the mind most effectually works on the body ... insomuch that it is most true which Plato saith in his Charmides: *omnia corporis mala ab animâ procedere*, all the mischiefs of the body proceed from the soul" (*Anatomy of Melancholy*, Pt. 1, Sec. 2, Mem. 3, Subs. 1, p. 165). Elsewhere Burton says that Plato and Cyprian blame the soul while others accuse the body (ibid., pt. 1, Sec. 2, Mem. 5, Subs. 1, p. 246).
145. *Amaltheum Lexicon*, p. 341. The regulation of a dying man's conscience, in order to permit religious euthanasia, was an important duty of the priest which, in seventeenth- and eighteenth-century France, sometimes conflicted with the aims of the medical attendant. On this subject see Henri Bremond, *Histoire littéraire du sentiment religieux en France*, Paris, 1932, vol. IX, Chap. V, "L'art de mourir", pp. 350–1.
146. *Encyclopædia Britannica*, 11th ed., 1910–11, art. Cornaro, Luigi. His was a very celebrated case. Further information regarding his ailments and curative regime, as well as the editions and translations of

his books may be found in Dezeimeris, Ollivier, Raige-Delorme, *Dictionnaire historique de la médecine ancienne et moderne*, Paris, 1828–39, 4 vols., vol. 1, pp. 864–5.

147. Pechlin, Obs. XX, p. 444.
148. See §21.
149. "... *ad nescio quem instinctum* ...".
150. See Gaub I, §86.
151. "... *conditiones secundam naturam* ..." (Gaub, *Institutiones*, §2, p. 1).
152. "... *praeter, aut contra naturam* ..." (ibid.).
153. Ibid., §3, pp. 1, 2.
154. "... *voluntate consciâ, et coeco instinctu* ..." (ibid., §4, p. 2).
155. Ibid., §6, p. 2.
156. Ibid., §51, p. 15.
157. "... *naturae humanae virtus pervigil* ..." (ibid.).
158. "... *naturam morborum medicatricem, medicum Naturae ministrum esse* ..." (ibid., §51, p. 16). See Note 162.
159. Ibid., §104, p. 33. "*Rara sine vulnere victoria*" (§105, p. 34).
160. "*Vocibus hi tantum, non re ipsâ, dissentiunt* ..." (ibid., §52, p. 17).
161. Ibid., §649, p. 254.
162. Ibid., §99, 100, pp. 31, 32. One of the best-known passages in the Hippocratic corpus is that in which the "natures" are called the physicians of disease, and some of the ways (tears, expectoration, coughing, etc.) in which untaught nature performs this task are mentioned (Hippocrates/Littré, vol. 5, p. 315).
163. Ibid., §633–6, pp. 246–8.
164. *Amaltheum Lexicon*, p. 599.
165. "*Hic ille tam salubris* pepasmos *quo conditiones noxiae eorum, quae morbum intentant aut faciunt, ita mitescunt, ut vel innocuae fiant, vel ad commodam ejectionem expeditae*" (Gaub, *Institutiones*, §637, p. 248).
166. Ibid.
167. Ibid., §638, p. 248.
168. "... *ut certius aliud potentiusve cum ad sanandos, tum ad praecavendos morbos auxilium natura, vel ars, vix agnoscat*" (ibid., §641, p. 249).
169. Ibid., §641, p. 249
170. Ibid., §643, 644, pp. 250, 251.
171. Ibid., §646, p. 252.
172. Boyle says that God has no need to play "after-games" in the universe, i.e. matter behaves in accordance with the laws of motion and no external agency, God, nature, or whatever intervenes (Robert Boyle, *Works*, London, 1772, Vol. 5, "A Free Inquiry into the Vulgarly Received Notion of Nature", pp. 162–3). He admits, however, the possible intervention of providence and the actual intervention of the rational soul or mind of man in these "hydraulico-pneumatical engines we call human bodies" (ibid., pp. 238–9).
173. Gaub, *Institutiones*, §647–9, pp. 252–4.

174. The prototype is the cosmic disturbance of "Chaos and old Night". Milton expresses it more literally than figuratively in the lines describing the "dark illimitable ocean" beyond the gates of hell,

> ... where eldest Night
> and Chaos, ancestors of Nature, hold
> Eternal anarchy, amidst the noise
> of endless wars, and by confusion stand.
> For Hot, Cold, Moist and Dry, four champions fierce,
> Strive here for mastery, and to battle bring
> Their embryon atoms: (*Paradise Lost*, Bk. II, 894–900).

This language of combat can also be found in Galen. The four qualities act on each other and are acted on in turn, the hot, cold, moist and dry, and of these there are two opposites, hot striving against cold and moist combating dry (Galen/Kühn, vol. I, *De temperamentis*, Bk. I, cap. 11, p. 518). The similarity of disturbances of physiological temperament—disturbances in balance of the qualities—and meteorological disturbances leads first to a characterization of the seasons of the year in terms of this balance and then to a relatively fixed relationship between the four chief temperaments and the four seasons. Galen, for example, in arguing against the viewpoint of the adherents of Athenaeus of Attalia, who claim that the hot and the moist together form a balanced temperament which does not give rise to disease, and likewise that spring, being hot and moist, is temperate (*eucratos*) whereas the three other seasons, summer, autumn and winter, being hot and dry, dry and cold, and cold and moist, respectively, are intemperate, agrees that these qualities go with the seasons but disagrees (for reasons that cannot detain us here) that the hot-moist temperament and the season of spring are perfectly balanced (ibid., cap. 111, iv, pp. 522–4). The writer of the pseudo-Galenical work *De humoribus* states, *Quod in mundo elementum id animalibus humor; quemadmodum et in anno tempestas*, adding that they are not exactly alike and going on to discuss the similarities and differences (Galen/Kühn, vol. XIX, pp. 485–96).

175. "... *restituto nervei generis tenore* ...".

176. *Amaltheum Lexicon*, p. 741.

177. Verhovitz, author of an eighteenth-century monograph on nostalgia, considered the disease a lesion of the imagination, curable only by a return home. He divided it into three varieties: idiopathic, complicated and simulated. The first, although associated with no other disease, may nevertheless give rise to a melancholy *cum materia* (i.e. with an organic component) or eventually prove fatal. The second is complicated by gastric, febrile and other disturbances (J. B. Friedrich, *Versuch einer Literargeschichte der Pathologie und Therapie der psychischen Krankheiten*, Würzburg, 1830, pp. 299–300). Baron Larrey

233

(1766–1842), inspector of health of the French armies under Napoleon, and later chief surgeon of the royal guard, discusses nostalgia at length in one of his memoirs. He believes that all affections of the mind, including the emotions, have their seat in the brain, and he attempts to explain nostalgia in terms of anatomical changes taking place in the brain from the beginning on. The desire to return home, which is the result of sensations transmitted to the brain by the sense organs produces a kind of expansion of the brain substance together with engorgement and slackness of the blood-vessels of the brain and its membranes. First the intellectual functions and then, as the disturbance moves more deeply into the brain, the motor functions suffer. In an attempt to bolster up his argument Larrey adduces clinical pictures similar to nostalgia but produced by head injury (*Recueil de mémoires de chirurgie, par le Baron D(ominique) J(ean) Larrey*, Paris, 1821, pp. 161–4). Troops from Holland, Switzerland and Breisgau are most susceptible to the "*impressions morales*" which lead to nostalgia, he remarks, and the condition was widespread during the Moscow campaign, but almost absent during the campaign in Egypt (ibid., pp. 168–9). Larrey's autopsy report on a patient dying with the diagnosis of nostalgia describes inflammation and suppuration of the meninges of the brain. He concludes that these patients do not die of gastro-enteritis, as has been believed, but as a result of changes taking place in the brain (ibid., pp. 168–9). Larrey gives various suggestions for preventing the onset of nostalgia (music, recreation, regular exercise, etc.) and states that it is up to "*la solicitude paternelle des chefs de corps éclairés par les lumières des chirurgiens-majors qu'appartient l'exécution des mesures indiquées ci-dessus pour prévenir la nostalgie, maladie d'autant plus grave qu'elle est insidieuse*" (ibid., p. 191).

178. Corp, pp. 85–93.
179. Johann Jakob Harder, *Dissertatio medica de nostalgia oder Heimweh, praeside Dn. Joh. Jac. Hardero, ad 22 Junium 1678, proponit Johannes Hoferus, Basileae*, p. 6. Harder (1656–1711) had just been appointed professor of rhetoric at the University of Basel, where he later obtained the chairs of anatomy and theoretical medicine.
180. Ibid., pp. 14, 15.
181. Zückert, pp. 59–60.
182. Corp, pp. 37–46. The physician who keeps hope alive in his patient has been censured for conduct "deemed improper in a religious view" (p. 41).
183. Ibid., p. 42.
184. *Diogenes Laertius, Lives of Eminent Philosophers, with an English translation by R. D. Hicks*, London, 1925, reprinted 1958, 2 vols., vol. 2, p. 453.
185. Corp, pp. 45–6.
186. Pechlin, Obs. XXVII, p. 464.

187. Ibid., Obs. XVI, p. 432.

188. Ibid., Obs. XXXV, p. 501.

189. In summing up these opinions Burton comments that toothache, gout, falling sickness and other maladies may be cured by words, charms and characters, yet . . . "All the world knows there is no virtue in such charms or cures, but a strong conceit and opinion alone. . . . The like we may say of our magical effects, superstitious cures, and such as are done by mountebanks and wizards. . . . An empirick oftentimes, and a silly chirurgion, doth more strange cures, than a rational physician. Nymannus gives a reason—because the patient puts his confidence in him; which Avicenna *prefers before all art, precepts, and all remedies whatsoever.* 'Tis opinion alone (saith Cardan) that makes or marrs physicians; and he doth the best cures, according to Hippocrates, in whom most trust" (*Anatomy of Melancholy*, Pt. 1, Sec. 2, Mem. 3, Subs. 2, p. 169). Roger Bacon has an interesting if conventional discussion of the subject. He considers that charms and signs are not to be wholly approved of, but that the skilled physician or whoever else has to arouse the soul (*anima*) may find it useful to apply them in order to give the patient confidence, hope and joy so that genuine remedies will be more eagerly and faithfully taken. If the physician does this without fraud and does not believe that the signs and charms are effective in themselves, the procedure is acceptable, *quoniam anima excitata potest in corpore proprio multa renovare, ut de infirmatate ad sanitatem convalescet, ex gaudio et confidentia.* He then cites Constantinus Africanus and Avicenna in support of this position, stating that in his *De anima* the latter holds the soul to be capable of exerting great power over its body by means of strong emotions (*Opera quaedam hactenus inedita*, London, 1859, pp. 527–8).

190. Pierre Gassendi, *Viri illustris Nicolai Fabricii de Peiresc, . . . Parisiis, 1641.*

191. Pechlin, Obs. XXVII, p. 466.

192. Valangin, p. 314. "Ramasini" is probably Bernardino Ramazzini (1633–1714), author of books on epidemiology and occupational diseases.

193. Hippocrates/Littré, vol. 8, p. 469.

194. Stahl/Gottlieb, p. 25.

195. Ibid., p. 26.

196. Valangin, pp. 336–7.

197. Boerhaave/van Eems, p. 479.

198. Ibid., p. 555.

199. Ibid., p. 482.

200. Corp, p. 3.

201. Zückert, pp. 12, 77, 78.

202. Smith, p. 199.

203. Ibid., p. 42.

204. Ibid., p. 43. Modern neurologists attempt to transform psychological disturbances into neurological disturbances in a rather similar way; Stewart Wolf, for example speaks of the power of the nervous system over the rest of the body and argues that all organs of the body are capable of responding to nervous stimuli arising from "meaningful" situations. For him, as for other "neurologizers" there is no real problem here, since the distinction between physical disease and mental disease is without meaning, the brain being a part of the physical organism and mental disease being in reality brain disease (Stewart Wolf, "Disease as a Way of Life: Neural Integration in Systemic Pathology", *Perspectives in Biology and Medicine*, IV: 288, 1961).

205. Boerhaave, *Institutiones*, §771, p. 387.

206. Elizabethan Galenical views may be found in Timothy Bright's *A Treatise of Melancholy* (Facsimile Text Society, New York, 1948) and in Robert Burton's *Anatomy of Melancholy*. Because of the ready accessibility of these two works and the more systematic treatment accorded to our topic in Thomas Wright's *Passions of the Minde in Generalle* (first published in 1601) I shall give its contents here in some detail, making use of the enlarged and revised edition of 1621. *Definition of the passions:* Wright accepts Damascene's eighth-century definition of the passions as sensual motions of the appetitive faculty due to the imagination of some good or ill thing (following lines with which we are familiar) and says that beasts and children, even before they acquire the use of reason, also have emotions. He quotes Augustine's words, which are worth requoting in order to show the uniformity of the Western tradition, as follows. The motions of the soul (*motus animae*) which the Greeks call *pathê* are called by certain Latins, as Cicero in the *Tusculan Disputations*, perturbations (*perturbationes*). Others call them affections (*affectiones*), others affects (*affectus*), and others expressly passions (*passiones*). Wright then justifies the use of these several terms and shows how intimately he conceives the emotions to be connected with bodily changes. Although they are *acts* of the appetitive faculty they are called *passions*, he says, because when stirring in the mind they *cause* a passion or alteration in the humors of the body (Descartes will later invert this causal sequence). They are called perturbations because they corrupt the judgement and seduce the will, and affections because "the soule by them, either affecteth some good, or for the affection of some good, detesteth some il(l)". The passions, then, are internal acts or operations of the soul, bordering on immaterial reason on one side and material sense on the other, "prosecuting some good thing, or flying some ill thing, causing therewithall some alteration in the body" (ibid., pp. 4, 5). *Classification of the emotions:* Aristotle reduces all passions to pleasure and pain, says Wright, and the "modern philosophers" who make the passions dependent on the procuring of something thought good or the avoidance of something

thought bad aim at almost the same mark, since we strive for pleasure in the one case and seek to avoid pain in the other. Wright follows the Thomists and places six passions in the coveting (*concupiscibilis*) appetite: love, desire, delight, hatred, abomination and sadness; five lie in the invading (*irascibilis*) appetite: hope, despair, fear, audacity, and ire. All of these passions, he repeats, are evident, sometimes even best exemplified, in animals. Another way of classifying the passions offered by Wright is of great physiological interest: they may be divided into those accompanied by dilatation, enlargement and "diffusion" of the heart, or by contraction, collection and compression—for in all passions the heart is either dilated or constricted (pp. 22–4). *The heart and the emotions:* The heart of a man changes his countenance, says Wright—and here a very fine line is drawn between the literal and figurative use of the word "heart"—for in anger or fear men become high colored or pale, whereas in sorrow their eyes are heavy and in joy lively. The passions alter the countenance in varying degree but reside elsewhere. The face is not the "root and core" but only the "rind and leaves" of the passions (pp. 27–30). The external actions are the signs of the internal passions, they are like windows through which a man must pass to discover the secret affections of another's heart (ibid., p. 172). In order to understand Wright properly we must not forget his conception of the "corporeality" of the passions. There may indeed, he writes, be passions, or something like them, in the highest part of the soul, completely divorced from corporeal substance, indeed the Scriptures ascribe love, hate and anger to God. But the "passions of the mind" are concerns of the sensitive and appetitive faculties and therefore border on corporeality. The "affections of the will", bred and born in the highest part of the soul, are immaterial, spiritual and independent of bodily instruments, but those of the appetites are material and corporeal to the extent that they require bodily instrumentation. As the powers of sight, hearing, smelling, tasting and touching have as their "corporeal instruments" the eyes, ears, nose, tongue and flesh, do the passions of the mind have a particular bodily organ with which they are bound up? To which Wright answers, the heart is that organ, in both men and beasts. He offers our everyday experience of the involvement of the heart in the passions—the heart is pained, constricted, heavy, and so on—in support of this belief. We prove in our hearts the workings of our passions, and "by the noise of their tumult we understand the work of their presence". The understanding has its seat in the brain, which is soft and otherwise fitted to receive the forms of objects; the heart is endowed with fiery spirits and is best fitted for affecting. When objects are present and possessed the passions can be said to involve the whole body, even though their seat remains in the heart. Wright accepts the belief that the humors move toward the heart during the arousal of the passions. He asks, to what end does this movement occur? God and Nature do not work by chance, or without giving rise to some benefit. The answer, he believes, is that the heart, although prepared by nature to digest the blood sent from the liver, does not always have the temperature (i.e. the mixture) required by the passions—love will have heat, sadness cold, fear constricts, and pleasure expands. As the efficient cause of the movement of the humors to the heart, he suggests a combined effect of "drawing" on part of the heart and the "expulsive virtue" of the part from whence the humors come (pp. 32–6). *The temperaments and the emotions:* We may confirm the old saying, *Animi mores corporis temperaturam sequantur* (a version of the title of Galen's well-known essay, which Wright translates as "the manners of the soule follow the temperature of the body"), by observing the characteristic differences of behavior in men of phlegmatic, choleric, melancholy and sanguine complexions (temperaments). There are characteristic differences of age groups and sexes. Young men are hot, incontinent and bold, old men are cold, covetous and cautious, women are envious, proud and inconstant, and so on (pp. 37–40). *Mechanism of the emotions:* Wright admits that the "motions of our passions" are hidden from our eyes, yet it is necessary to speculate on the matter and he offers the following scheme. The imagination, or internal sense, and consequently the passions, are aroused in three ways: by humors arising in the body, by the external senses, and by the command of reason (p. 149). In the second case some known object is presented to the imagination (which resides in the forepart of the brain). This object must be "known" before we can fear or desire it. Then "purer spirits" move by "certaine secret channels" to the heart where they signify the object, whether convenient or inconvenient. The heart then bends to seek or avoid that object, and in so doing draws to itself humors from other parts of the body—in pain and sadness melancholy blood, in anger, blood and choler, and so on. When we feel hunger in our stomachs the same soul that informs the stomach resides also in the hands, eyes and mouth, and subordinates them to serve the stomach and satisfy its need. Just so in the "hunger of the heart", the spleen, liver, blood spirits, choler and melancholy attend and serve that organ diligently (pp. 45–46). *How the emotions alter the body:* Moderate joy promotes the health, says Wright, because the "purer spirits" retire to the heart and help in the digestion of blood. This produces an abundance of spirits which are then sent to all parts of the body, both causing a good concoction and helping in the expulsion of superfluities. This, in turn, leads to a good color, good countenance, and universal bodily health. If this emotion is too strong, however, the heart becomes hot and inflamed due to the continual abundance of "spirit" and in consequence it generates "cholericke and burned blood" (the "adust" humors spoken of by writers of this period). In addition, excessive joy dilates the heart and

238

may lead to sudden death.   Yet the passions which constrict the heart—fear, sadness, despair—are far more dangerous to the body.   Many men have lost their lives from sadness and fear, says Wright, but few from love and hope.   The effects exerted by passions of this kind are due to an accumulation of melancholy blood about the heart.   By interfering with the digestion of blood additional melancholy humor is produced which, because it is cold and dry, tends to extinguish the two qualities most important to life, heat and moisture.   Few men, says Wright, are not at times subject to melancholy humors that trouble their minds and bodies.   The passions that constrict the heart initiate some diseases and make all of them worse.   Passions engender humors, on the one hand, and humors breed passions on the other.   The state of the humors depends in turn on external causes: air, sleep, waking, meat, drink, exercise and rest (ibid., pp. 59–65).   Every vehement passion alters some of the humors of the body, and all physicians agree that among the different causes of disease one—and that not the least—is an excess of passion (p. 4).   (This is, of course, the doctrine of the non-naturals, although Wright does not use the term.)   *The mind-body problem:* I could propound a hundred questions about the soul and body, says Wright toward the end of his book, which are disputed over by divines, physicians, and natural and moral philosophers.   He does in fact propound one hundred and twenty such questions.   Some of them concern the problem of extension.   How can the soul, being a spirit indivisible and without extension, extend itself throughout the body? What happens to the soul informing a bodily part when that part is cut off?   Other aspects of the mind-body problem appear in one form or another.   How can the will command a toe or arm to move, and presently it does?   How do the corporeal humors of the body stir up the passions and the passions in turn generate corporeal humors? How can a corporeal imagination concur with a spiritual conceit? (pp. 298, 299, 304).   The last question is particularly interesting in connection with a similar distinction later to be drawn by Descartes with respect to the corporeal substance of an image in the brain and our awareness of this image, and requires some explanation.   The power of forming images, whether of external objects or of things conceived internally, Wright calls the "imagination".   These images are, to Wright (just as they were later to Descartes), corporeal events taking place in a definite part of the brain.   A "conceit" on the other hand is a spiritual, incorporeal, apprehension of the mind, a conception, that is. The problem is again one of relating two disparate realms, and the solution is attempted with the aid of intermediaries, the passions.   We can see this in Wright's answer to the question: How possibly can a man's conceit work changes in his body? (p. 65).   Hippocrates, says Wright, advised physicians to give their patients the meat they preferred even though it might be a little more harmful than meat not so well liked. Philosophers and physicians all agree that the patient's opinion of the physician's abilities and the virtues of the remedies proffered is of great importance in effecting the cure of any malady. The reason is that the imagination herein (i.e. the corporeal events corresponding to the "spiritual conceit") arouses the passions of hope and pleasure. These in turn arouse the "purer spirits" which, cooperating with Nature, strengthen her in the performance of any corporeal action or vital function (p. 66). We gain additional insight into Wright's difficulties with the mind-body problem if we briefly consider his reflections on a question borrowed from Augustine, as difficult as any in natural and moral philosophy according to Wright. How does music stir up the passions and affections? What has a shaking or wave-like motion of the air—the substance of music—to do with arousing lust, anger, pleasure, and religious devotion? It is not so remarkable, he says, that meat, drink, exercise and so forth stir up the passions, since it is clear that they alter the humors, but how can simple sounds do this as well? Wright is unable to resolve the problem; he can only point to a certain sympathy between our souls and music, as inexplicable as that between the loadstone and the needle, and suggest that the wave-like motion is transmitted to the heart where it plays on the vital and animal spirits that are the instruments and spurs of the passions (pp. 168–70).

207. In view of his key position in the history of medicine as the discoverer of the accepted mode of circulation of the blood and the inaugurator of modern physiology the handful of references to the emotions scattered through Harvey's writings are of great interest, and it is most unfortunate that no trace of the "Observations", where, as he remarks in his second essay to Riolan, these matters are unravelled and clarified, has ever been found (Harvey/Franklin, p. 165). Harvey agrees that sorrow, love, hate and other emotions may cause wasting, humoral derangement and "multiple indigestions" which form the prelude to diseases and fatalities. His explanation is that every affection of the mind with sorrow, joy, hope or anxiety changes the temper, pulsation and other features of the heart, polluting all ingesta, weakening the bodily powers and sometimes giving rise to incurable disease in the body (Harvey/Franklin, *Movement of the Heart and Blood*, Ch. 15, p. 89–90). The digested food must be received, perfected and distributed to the members of the body, and the heart is the site of this process. The heart is the forceful agent necessary for the distributive process, since blood tends naturally to move to a concentration point—cold, fear, horror and the like cause this to occur rapidly (ibid., p. 90). Again, in the second essay to Riolan, Harvey remarks that when a frightened patient faints during venesection we see that the surface of the body becomes pallid; this is due to the immediate cessation of the outward flow of blood. So many possibilities at once suggest themselves, writes Harvey, that another treatise would be required. For what is more remarkable than the way

in which the body reacts to every emotion and appetite—the eyes redden, the pupils are constricted, in bashfulness the cheeks blush, in fear or shame the face is pale, in adolescents touched with desire the penis is at once filled with blood, erected and extended (ibid., "Second Essay", p. 165). For Harvey's comments on the effects of anger see Gaub II, Note 74.

208. "... *ob retentas a partu secundas in aphoniam incidit* ...".

209. *Amaltheum Lexicon*, p. 433. In discussing hysteria Galen suggests the retention of menstrua or seed as causes: "... *ob retenta menstrua vel semen cohibitum* ... *ob seminis retentionem utpote quod magnam vim obtinent et in mulieribus humidius ac frigidius sit et excretionem requirat* ..." (Galen/Kühn, vol. VIII, *De locis affectis* VI, v, p. 417).

210. Agrippa von Nettesheim recounts the story of Alexander the Great (*lumen et ignem ex se profundere*) and adds that the father of Theodoric, under similar circumstances, gave off sparks (*ignis scintillas ex toto corpore profudisse*) but where Gaub found the story I do not know (Agrippa, cap. lxiii, pp. 101–2).

211. *Attic Nights*, V, ix.

212. "Willius" is probably Johann Valentin Wille, whose dissertation, *De ira*, was published in 1691. "Robinson" may be Nicholas Robinson (1697–1795), the author of *A New System of the Spleen, Vapours and Hypochondriac Melancholy* ..., London, 1729 (Hunter and Macalpine, pp. 342–7; see also Note 29). For Borrichius see Gaub I, 83.

213. Zückert, p. 51.

214. Corp, p. 56.

215. Corp, p. 55; Zückert, p. 50.

216. Pechlin, Obs. XXVI, pp. 460–3.

217. Corp, pp. 60, 61.

218. Ibid., p. 62.

219. "*Mentis alienationes cujusmodicunque, furiosas, hystericas, hypochondriacas, febriles* ...".

220. Gaub can hardly have been unacquainted with Sydenham's observations on hysteria, in view of Boerhaave's extremely high opinion of Sydenham, whom he called the one physician of modern times worthy to be compared with Hippocrates.

221. *Thomas Sydenham, The Works, translated from the Latin edition of Dr. Greenhill by R. C. Latham, M.D.*, 2 vols., London, 1852, vol. 2, Letter to Dr. Cole, pp. 84 et seq. A very detailed historical study of hysteria may be found in Glafira Abricossoff, *L'Hystérie aux XVIIe et XVIIIe siècles* (thesis), Paris, 1897. The earliest references to "hysteria" are in the Hippocratic writings—the uterus is the cause of a thousand ills, says Democritus (Hippocrates/Littré, vol. 9, p. 397) in a passage cited by Sydenham in his Letter to Dr. Cole. Various clinical pictures thought to be dependent on the site and direction of uterine displacement, many of which are recognizable as hysteria,

may be found in the Hippocratic treatise on diseases of women (Hippocrates/Littré, vol. 8, pp. 33–5, 257–79).

222. *Amaltheum Lexicon*, p. 433.
223. Boerhaave/van Eems, pp. 481–2.
224. Smith, p. 165.
225. Laroque, p. 16.
226. "*Quamobrem et apparatu opus est, qui vehementissime perterreat, et submersione tam diuturna totiesque iterata, ut vita reapse in discrimen adducatur, dubiumque sit, utrum omnino perierit retractus, anne queat reviviscere: secus enim certae opis nihil expectandum.*"
227. Franciscus Mercurius van Helmont, *The spirit of disease, or diseases from the spirit: laid open in some observations concerning man and his diseases. Wherein is shewed how much the mind influenceth the body in causing and curing of diseases*, London, 1694, pp. 43–48, cited from Hunter and Macalpine, pp. 254–5.
228. Robert Boyle, *Works*, London, 1744, vol. 5, "Of the usefulness of natural philosophy"; Pt. II, Sec. I, "Of its usefulness to physick", Essay V, Chap. X, pp. 527–8. The Salmuth referred to is probably Philipp, author of the posthumously published book, *P. Salmuthi observationum medicarum . . .*, Braunschweig, 1648.
229. Ibid., *Works*, London, 1772, vol. 5, "A Free Inquiry into the Vulgarly Received Notion of Nature", p. 199. Boyle makes only one reference to the non-naturals as such in this essay—"the six non-natural things so much spoken of by physicians" (ibid., p. 220). This is almost exactly Burton's phrase—"those six non-natural things, so much spoken of amongst physicians" (*Anatomy of Melancholy*, Pt. 1, Sec. 2, Mem. 2, Subs. 1, p. 140).
230. Pechlin, Obs. XXII, pp. 447–9.
231. Ibid., Obs. XXIV, p. 453.
232. Ibid., Obs. XXIV, p. 454.
233. Stahl/Gottlieb, p. 33.
234. Boerhaave/van Eems, pp. 414, 415.
235. Ibid., p. 415.
236. Valangin, p. 234.
237. Juncker, p. 235.
238. Corp, pp. 73–7.
239. Ibid., pp. 80, 81.
240. Ibid., pp. 82, 83.
241. M. Weikard, *Der philosophische Arzt, neue Auflage*, 3 vols., Frankfurt/M., 1798, vol. 3, pp. 263–4. Weikard was personal physician to Catherine the Great from 1784 to 1789.
242. Ibid., p. 269.
243. Boerhaave/van Eems, p. 413.
244. *Attic Nights*, XIX, xii.
245. *Tusculan Disputations*, II, xxv.

Appendix I

The following editions and translations of Jerome Gaub's *De regimine mentis* were used in the preparation of the present book.

1. *Sermo academicus de regimine mentis quod medicorum est.... Lugduni Batavorum, apud Balduinum van der Aa,* 1747. Bound with *Sermo academicus alter de regimine mentis ... Lugduni Batavorum, apud Samuelem et Joannem Luchtmans,* 1763.

2. *Sermo academicus de regimine mentis ... editio altera, Lugduni Batavorum, apud Cornelium de Pecker,* 1767. Bound with *Sermo academicus alter de regimine mentis ... Lugduni Batavorum, apud Samuelem et Joannem Luchtmans,* 1763.

3. *Sermo academicus de regimine mentis ... editio altera, Lugduni Batavorum, apud Cornelium de Pecker,* 1767. Bound with *Sermo academicus alter de regimine mentis ... editio altera, Lugduni Batavorum, apud Samuelem et Joannem Luchtmans,* 1769.

4. *Sermones II. academici de regimine mentis ... editio tertia prioribus accuratior, Argentorati, ex oficina libraria Amandi König,* 1776.

5. *Von der Regierung des Geistes welche den Aerzten zukommt* (anon., n.p., n.d.). (A translation of the second essay only, probably made in the eighteenth century.)

6. *On the Passions; or, A Philosophical Discourse Concerning the Duty and Office of Physicians in the Management and Cure of Diseases of the Mind....* Translated by J. Taprell, London (n.d.). (A translation of the first essay only, probably made in the eighteenth century.)

7. *De regimine mentis, orationes duo—Zwei akademische Reden über die heilkundliche Wirkung der Seele, Opuscula selecta Neerlandicorum,* vol. XI, Amsterdam, 1932. (Contains a German translation by L. Hellman based on a Dutch translation of 1775 by W. Servaas.)

The editions of the first essay are *princeps* (1747), *altera* (1767) and *tertia* (1776); of the second essay, *princeps* (1763) *altera* (1769), *tertia* (1776). The texts of the first editions of both essays were reset and reprinted in volume XI of the *Opuscula selecta Neerlandicorum* (Amsterdam, 1932). In the table below P stands for *princeps*, A for *altera*, T for *tertia* and RP for the reprint. The paragraphs are those of the first editions. The texts of all editions are substantially the same. There are numerous typographical errors, however. I have italicized what seem to me the correct readings and suggested one minor emendation of the text (in parenthesis).

Essay I

Para.	4	P, A, RP,	*tantummodo*	T, tantummode
	8	P, A, RP	*humanae*	T, humane
	9	P, A, RP	*quoque*	T, quoqne
	13	P, A, RP	*observatio*	T, obsorvatio
	18	P, A, RP	*facilitas*	T, facillitas
	37	P, A, RP	*unum*	T, ounum
		P, A, RP	*temporis*	T, remporis
	41	P, A, RP	*exercentur*	T, ererentur
	47	P, A, RP	*illud*	T, jllud
	61	P, A, RP	*tandem*	T, tanden
	76	P, A, RP	*proficient*	T, profic ent
	94	P, A, RP	*componant*	T, componat
	13	P, A, T	*videre*	RP, vivere
	35	P, A, T	*convitium*	RP, conventium
	61	P, A	Ctharaginensium	T, Cartharaginensium
				RP, *Carthaginensium*
	96	P, T, RP	*apparuit*	A, appatuit

Essay II

Para.	3	P, A, RP	*meditatione*	T, meditaione
	4	P, RP	ignorati	A, T, *ignorari*
	17	P, A, RP	*narrando*	T, rarando
	29	P, A, RP	*adamussim*	T, ad amussim
	34	P, A, RP	*quae*	T, que
		P, RP	benificentia	A, T, *beneficientia*
	36	P, RP	mereatur	A, T, mereatut
		P, A, RP	audace	T, *audaci*

41	P, RP	plus dicam	A, period missing from sentence preceding "plus dicam"
			T, "plus dicam" displaced to preceding sentence
8	P, A, T	*fiducia*	RP, siducia
15	P, A, T	*figmenta*	RP, sigmenta
28	P, A, T	*fucum*	RP, sucum
30	P, A, T	*probari*	RP, provari
	P, A, T	*quibus infirmi*	RP, quibusinfirmi
33	P, A, T	*alia atque alia*	RP, alia atque
	P, A, T	*inconsiderate*	RP, inconsideratae
36	P, A, T	*refutari*	RP, resutari
37	P, A, T	*gravi*	RP, oravi
38	P, A, T	*ostenderim*	RP, stenderim
	P, A, T	*frigidos*	RP, erigidos
41	P, A, T	*fulcris* (twice)	RP, sulcris (twice)
42	P, A, T	*cum jam*	RP, cumi am
	P, A, T	*adducatur*	RP, adducator
	P, A, T	*caeli*	RP, calli
47	P, A, T	*ne*	RP, de
	P, T,	*omnifariae*	A, multifariae
			RP, omnivariae
	P, A, T	*ob*	RP, op
23	P, A	cottidiani	T, cortidiani
			RP, *cotidiani*
34	P, A	quantocyus	T, quanto ocyus
			RP, *quantocius*
	P, A, T, RP	gnavo	(*gnaro*)

The emendation, *gnaro* for *gnavo*, in the sentence, *Verum rudissimus quisque cum sciente, stupidus cum gnavo, infans cum adulto commune habet*, is perhaps questionable, but *gnarus* fits the sequence of antitheses where *gnavus* does not. Gaub's anonymous eighteenth-century German translator evidently thought so as well, since he renders *stupidus cum gnavo* as *der Thörigste mit dem Weisen*, and Hellman's translation from the Dutch reads similarly.

Appendix II

The translation has been made as literal as possible within the bonds imposed by clarity and readability. I have neither attempted to reproduce the style and idiom of eighteenth-century English, nor to replace Gaub's long Latin sentences with shorter equivalents in modern English. The result is a heavily Latinized English containing a few archaisms and outmoded rhetorical devices. Certain problems arising in connection with the translation require comment at this point. In the first essay Gaub uses the word *animus* seventy-four times, and in the second eighty-five times. *Mens* appears eighty-three times in the first, and nineteen in the second. For the most part he uses the two terms interchangeably, and I have usually translated both as "mind". Gaub writes, for example, of the *animi facultates* and the *mentis facultates* (faculties of the mind) with no obvious difference in meaning. The *animi potestates* and the *mentis potestates* (powers of the mind) appear in the same context, as do the *regimen mentis* and the *regimen animi* (management of the mind). In two instances (I, 18; II, 41) I have rendered *animus* as "soul" for idiomatic reasons; in both the phrase *toto animo* is used. The word "soul" occurs in only one other passage (I, 84), where it is a translation of *anima* in the phrase *de aeterno animae suae salute*, the Christian soul clearly being meant. On one occasion (I, 30), in connection with the words *de summa illa animi firmitate*, the word *animus* has been translated as "spirit". The word "spirit" occurs three times again, in I, 18, I, 78 and II, 7, as a translation of *ingenium*. The phrases *motus animi* and *perturbationes animi* are well-recognized equivalents of what were formerly called the "passions" and are now called the "emotions". Gaub never uses the phrase *motus mentis*, and the phrase *perturbatam mentem* occurs only once (II, 14) and in a context suggesting that it is antonymous with *tranquillam mentem* (II, 30), hence I have translated the one phrase as "disturbed mind" and the other as "tranquil mind". *Motus animi* and *perturbatio animi* have been translated as "emotion" throughout, with three exceptions, even though "emotional disturbance" might convey the meaning better to a modern reader unfamiliar with the older view that *all* emotions are disturbances of the mind. The three exceptions occur in I, 82 and II, 47, where "disturbance in the mind" and "emotional disturbances" appear, and in I, 90, where *animi motus* is translated as "emotional disturbance". The phrase *commotus animus* occurs twice (I, 26; II, 16) and has been translated as "disturbed mind" in both instances. The phrase *commotio animi* has been translated as "emotion" on one occasion (II, 36), and as "emotional disturbance" on two (II, 41, 42) in accordance with the demand of the context. Occurring alone on two occasions (II, 16; II, 48) and qualified by *animus* on a third (I, 71) *affectio* has been translated as "affection". *Affectus* occurs twice (I, 78; II, 48) and has been translated as "affection" in both instances. The reader will also observe that while the usual pronoun for "mind" is "it", in a few instances I have used the pronoun "she" in order to avoid ambiguity. Finally, Gaub uses a Greek term, *pathê*, in II, 40, which I have translated as "emotions".

Bibliography of Books and Papers Cited in the Introduction, Commentaries and Notes

(See also Appendix I)

A. BOOKS

ABRICOSSOFF, GLAFIRA, *L'Hystérie aux XVIIe et XVIIIe siècles* (*thesis*), Paris, 1897.

AGRIPPA VON NETTESHEIM, HENRY CORNELIUS, *De occulta philosophia* .... *Lugduni, per Beringos fratres*, n.d., 2 vols.

ALPINI, PROSPERO, *De praesagienda vita et morti aegrotantium libri septem* ... *cum praefatione Hermanni Boerhaave. Editio altera Leidensis, cujus textum recensuit, passim emendavit, supplevit; citata Hippocratis loca accuravit, Hieron. Dav. Gaubius*, Lugduni Batavorum ... 1733.

Amaltheum Castello-Brunonianum, sive Lexicon Medicum, Patavii, 1746.

ANON., "Eloge de M. Gaubius", *Histoire de la société royale de médecine, année 1779*, Paris, 1782.

ARNOLD, MAGDA, *Emotion and Personality*, New York, 1960, 2 vols.

AVICENNA, *Cantica Avicennae a magistro Armengaudo Blash de Montepesulano ex arabico in latinum translata, cum castigationibus clarissimi philosophi ac medici Andreae Bellunensis* (*in liber canonis*), Venice, 1555.

AVICENNA, *Liber canonis* ... *a Gerardo Carmonensi ex arabico sermone in latinum conversa*, Venice, 1555.

BACON, ROGER, *Opera quaedam hactenus inedita*, London, 1859.

BLEULAND, JAN B., *Oratio qua memoria Hieronymi Davidis Gaubii cum omnibus tum praesertim medicina studiosus commendatur*, Harderwyck, 1792.

BOAS, GEORGE, "Some Problems of Intellectual History", (in) *Studies in Intellectual History*, Johns Hopkins, 1953 (source of citation on p. v., pp. 14, 15).

BOERHAAVE, HERMANN, *Institutiones medicae, digestae ab Hermanno Boerhaave, ed. Leydensis sexta*, Lugduni Batavorum, 1746.

BOERHAAVE, HERMANN, *Opera omnia medica, oratio II, de usu ratiocinii mechanici in medicina habita in auditorio magno 24 Septembris, a. 1702*, Venice, 1747.

Boerhaave, Hermann, *Praelectiones Academicae de Morbis Nervorum, quas ex auditorum manuscriptis collectas edi curavit Jacobus van Eems, medicus Leydensis,* Lugduni Batavorum, 1761. Referred to as "Boerhaave/van Eems".

Boyle, Robert, *The Sceptical Chymist,* 1661, reprinted London, 1949.

Boyle, Robert, *Works,* London, 1772, 5 vols.

Bremond, Henri, *Histoire littéraire du sentiment religieux en France,* Paris, 1932.

Bright, Timothy, *A Treatise of Melancholy,* Facsimile Text Society, New York, 1948.

Buchanan, Scott, *The Doctrine of Signatures, A Defence of Theory in Medicine,* London, 1938.

Burton, Robert, *Anatomy of Melancholy,* 16th ed., London, 1936.

Cabanis, Pierre Jean George, *Coup d'œil sur les révolutions et sur la réforme de la médecine,* (in) *Œuvres Philosophiques,* Presses Universitaires de France, 1956, 2 vols.

Cannon, Walter, *The Wisdom of the Body,* revised and enlarged edition 1939, reprinted 1963, New York.

Carrère, Joseph, *Dissertatio medica de vitali corporis et animae foedere,* Perpignan, 1758.

Celsus, *De medicina, with an English translation by W. G. Spencer,* London, 1928, 3 vols.

Chauvet, Emmanuel, *La philosophie des médecins grecs,* Paris, 1886.

Cicero, *De Oratore, with an English translation by H. Rackham,* London, 1942, reprinted 1960, 2 vols.

Cicero, *The Speeches, with an English translation by N. H. Watts,* London, 1923.

Cicero, *Tusculan Disputations, with an English translation by J. E. King,* London, 1927, revised and reprinted 1960.

Collingwood, R. G., *Metaphysics,* Oxford, 1940.

Corp, *An Essay on the Changes Produced in the Body by the Operations of the Mind, by the late Doctor Corp of Bath,* London, 1791.

Daremberg, Charles H., *Œuvres de Galien,* Paris, 1854, 2 vols.

Descartes, René, *Œuvres et Lettres,* Librairie Gallimard, Paris, 1953. (All citations of Descartes have been taken from this complete edition of his works in French.) Referred to as "Descartes".

Dezeimeris, Ollivier, Raige-Delorme, *Dictionnaire historique de la médecine ancienne et moderne,* Paris, 1828–39, 4 vols.

DIELS, HERMANN, *Die Fragmente der Vorsokratiker, Griechisch und Deutsch*, 7te Aufl., hrsg. W. Kranz, Berlin, 1954, 3 vols.

ECCLES, JOHN, *The Neurophysiological Basis of Mind*, Oxford, 1953.

EDELSTEIN, LUDWIG, *The Hippocratic Oath* (Supplements to the *Bulletin of the History of Medicine*, 1), Baltimore, 1943.

EISLER, RUDOLF, *Wörterbuch der Philosophischen Begriffe*, 2te Aufl., Berlin, 1904, 2 vols.

FASCH, AUGUSTIN, *Disputatio inauguralis medica de autocheiria praeside Dn. Augustino Henrico Faschio . . . subjicit Fredericus Hoffmanus, Jenae*, 31 Jan. 1681.

FEUCHTERSLEBEN, ERNST VON, *The Principles of Medical Psychology*, translated by H. E. Lloyd, London, 1847.

FORCELLINI, AEGIDIUS, *Totius latinitatis lexicon*, 3rd ed., Schneeberg, 1833, 4 vols.

FREEMAN, KATHLEEN, *Ancilla to the Pre-Socratic Philosophers*, Oxford, 1952.

FRERICHS, FRIEDRICH THEODOR, *Klinik der Leberkrankheiten*, Braunschweig, 1858, 2 vols.

FRIEDREICH, J. B., *Versuch einer Literargeschichte der Pathologie und Therapie der psychischen Krankheiten*, Würzburg, 1830.

GASSENDI, PIERRE, *Viri illustris Nicolai Fabricii de Peiresc, . . .* Paris, 1641.

GAUB, JEROME, *Institutiones Pathologiae Medicinalis*, ed. alt., Leiden, 1775. Referred to, after initial citation, as "*Institutiones*".

GAUB, JEROME, *Libellus de methodo concinnandi formulas medicamentorum, editio altera revisa et aucta*, Lugduni Batavorum, 1752.

GAUB, JEROME, *Oratio de vana vitae longae, a chemicis promissae, exspectatione, Leidae*, 1734.

GAUB, JEROME, *Oratio qua ostenditur chemiam artibus academicis jure esse inserendam*, Lugduni Batavorum, 1731.

GAUB, JEROME, *Specimen inaugurale medicum exhibens ideam generalem solidarum corporis humani partium . . . ex auctoritate magnifici rectoris D. Joannis Ortwini Westenbergii . . . pro gradu doctoratus submittit Hieronymus David Gaubius, Heydelb. Palatin . . . 24 Augusti. 1725 . . .* Lugduni Batavorum . . . 1725.

GAUB, JOAN, *Johannis Gaubii epistola problematica . . . ad virum clarissimum Fredericum Ruyschium . . .* Amstelaedami, 1724.

GELLIUS, *The Attic Nights of Aulus Gellius, with an English translation by John C. Rolfe*, London, 1927, revised and reprinted, 1961, 3 vols.

GRAFENBERG, SCHENCK VON, *Observationum medicarum rararum, novarum, admirabilium et monstrosarum volumen,* Frankfort, 1602.

GRUNER, CHRISTIAN GOTTFRIED, *Anfangsgründe der medizinischen Krankheitslehre,* Linz, 1785 (a translation of Gaub's *Institutiones* with a brief biography).

GRUNER, O. C., *A Treatise on the Canon of Medicine of Avicenna, incorporating a translation of the first book,* London, 1930.

GUTSCH, KARL, *Die Schrift des Hieronymus David Gaub, De regimine mentis quod medicorum est, Inaugural Dissertation von Karl Gutsch, Referent Prof. Dr. Martin Müller,* München, 1939.

HALLER, ALBRECHT, *Epistolarum ab eruditis viris ab Alb. Hallerum scriptarum,* Berne, 6 vols., 1773–75.

HALLIE, PHILIP P., *Maine de Biran, Reformer of Empiricism 1766–1824,* Cambridge, 1959.

Handbuch der Geschichte der Medizin, ed. by Max Neuburger and Julius Pagel, Leipzig, 1902–05, 3 vols.

HARDER, JOHANN JAKOB, *Dissertatio medica de nostalgia oder Heimweh, praeside Dn. Joh. Jac. Hardero, ad 22 Junium 1678, proponit Johannes Hoferus, Basileae.*

HARTMANN, EDUARD VON, *Philosophy of the Unconscious, translation of the 9th edition of 1884,* London, 1931.

Harvey, William, The Circulation of the Blood and Other Writings, translated by Kenneth J. Franklin, London, 1963.

HAUKE, ERIKA, *Galen: Dass die Vermögen der Seele eine Folge der Mischungen des Körpers sind* (Abhandlungen zur Geschichte der Medizin und Naturwissenschaften, Heft 21), Berlin, 1937.

Hippocrates, with an English translation by W. H. S. Jones, Loeb Library, Cambridge, 1952, 4 vols.

HOLLAND, PHILIP, *Dissertatio medica inauguralis, pauca de mente in corpus effectibus, exponens . . . ex auctoritate D. Gulielmi Robertson . . . subjicit Phillipus Holland,* Edinburgh, 1782.

HOOK, SYDNEY (ed.), *Dimensions of Mind,* New York, 1960.

HORST, GREGOR, *Marcellus Donatus, editio nova, De medica historia mirabili,* Frankfort, 1664.

HUME, DAVID, *An Enquiry Concerning Human Understanding* (reprint of posthumous edition of 1777), La Salle, 1952.

HUME, DAVID, *A Treatise of Human Nature* (reprinted from edition of London, 1739), London, 1955.

HUNTER, RICHARD AND MACALPINE, IDA, *Three Hundred Years of Psychiatry,* London, 1963.

JAEGER, WERNER, *Paideia: the Ideals of Greek Culture*, translated by Gilbert Highet, Oxford, 1944, 3 vols.

JAMES, WILLIAM, *Principles of Psychology*, New York, 1890, 2 vols.

JAUREGG, JULIUS WAGNER VON, *Die progressive Paralyse*, Neue Deutsche Klinik, Berlin, 1932, vol. 9.

JOANNITIUS (HUNAIN IBN ISHĀQ), *Isagoge ad tegni Galeni*, Leipzig, 1497.

JUNCKER, JOHANN, *Dissertatio inauguralis medica de noxa atque utilitate animi pathematum seu adfectuum in medicina, praeside Dn. Joanne Junckero, Auctor Ioanness Godofriedus Grunou*, Berlin, 1745.

KOESTLER, ARTHUR, *The Sleepwalkers*, New York, 1959, reprinted 1963.

KRETSCHMER, ERNST, *Körperbau und Character*, 5te und 6te Auflage, Berlin, 1926.

KRUMBHAAR, E. B., *Pathology*, New York, 1937.

KÜHN, C. G., *Claudii Galeni Opera Omnia*, Leipzig, 1821–33, 20 vols. Referred to as "Galen/Kühn".

LAEHR, HEINRICH, *Die Literatur der Psychiatrie, Neurologie und Psychologie im 18ten Jahrhundert*, Berlin, 1895.

LAERTIUS, DIOGENES, *Lives of Eminent Philosophers, with an English translation by R. D. Hicks*, London, 1925, reprinted 1958, 2 vols.

LAIN-ENTRALGO, PEDRO, *Heilkunde in geschichtlicher Entscheidung* (translated from the Spanish by Theodor Sapper), Vienna, 1956.

LAIN-ENTRALGO, PEDRO, *La Curación por la Palabra en la Antigüedad Clásica*, Madrid, 1958.

LAROQUE, RAIMUND, *De l'influence des passions sur l'économie animale, considérée dans les quatre âges de la vie.* Collections des thèses soutenues a l'école de Montpellier en l'an V et l'an VI, Montpellier, l'an VI.

LARREY, DOMINIQUE JEAN, *Recueil de mémoires de chirurgie, par le Baron D. Larrey*, Paris, 1821.

LEIBBRAND, WERNER, and WETTLEY, ANNEMARIE, *Der Wahnsinn: Geschichte der abendländischen Psychopathologie*, Freiburg/München, 1961.

LEIBNIZ, GOTTFRIED WILHELM, *Opera philosophica quae exstant latina gallica germanica*, 1959, Scientia, Aalen, 1959. All citations of Leibniz taken from this edition.

LEMNIUS, LEVINUS, *De habitu et constitutione corpore, quam Graeci krasin, triuiales complexionem vocant, Libri II* ... Frankfort, 1596.

LEMNIUS, LEVINUS, *The Touchstone of the Complexions ... fyrst wrytten in Latine, by Leuine Lemnie, and now Englished by Thomas Newton* ... London, 1581.

LITTRÉ, EMILE, *Œuvres complètes d'Hippocrate*, Paris, 1849, réimpression Amsterdam, 1962, 10 vols.

LOVEJOY, ARTHUR O., *The Revolt against Dualism*, La Salle, 1955.

MCDOUGALL, WILLIAM, *Body and Mind*, 1911, reprinted Boston, 1961.

MERCER, GRAEMIUS, *Dissertatio physico-medica inauguralis de pathematibus animi eorumque in corpus humanum effectibus ... ex auctoritate D. Gulielmi Robertson ... subjicit Graemius Mercer*, Edinburgh, 1784.

MERLEAU-PONTY, MAURICE, *The Phenomenology of Perception*, translated from the French by Colin Smith, London, 1962.

Minnesota Studies in the Philosophy of Science, vol. II, Concepts, Theories, and the Mind-Body Problem, edited by Herbert Feigl, Michael Scriven and Grover Maxwell, University of Minnesota, 1958.

MONTAIGNE, MICHEL DE, *Essais, texte établi et annoté par Albert Thibaudet*, Paris, 1950.

MORGAGNI, G. B., *The Seats and Causes of Diseases investigated by anatomy ... translated from the Latin of John Baptist Morgagni ... by Benjamin Alexander, M.D.*, London, 1769, 3 vols., facsimile ed., New York, 1960.

MUELLER, FERNAND-LOUIS, *Histoire de la psychologie de l'antiquité à nos jours*, Paris, 1960.

MURRAY, MARGARET A., *The Witch Cult in Modern Europe*, London, 1921, reprinted 1962.

NORDENSKIÖLD, ERIK, *The History of Biology ... translated from the Swedish by Leonard Bucknall Eyre*, New York, 1928.

PAULI, JOHANN, *Disputatio medica inauguralis de animi commotionum vi medica ... praeside Dn. Johanne Wilhelmo Pauli ... submittit Christianus Mentz*, 30 April 1700, Lipsiae.

PECHLIN, J. N., *Observationum physico-medicarum libri tres*, Hamburg, 1691.

PERDULCIS, BARTHOLOMEW, *De morbis animi*, Paris, 1639.

Plato, Charmides, translated by W. R. M. Lamb, Loeb Classical Library, London, 1955.

Plato, Timaeus, translated by R. G. Bury, London, 1952.

Plato, *The Collected Dialogues*, New York, 1963.

PLUTARCH, *Plutarch's Moralia, with an English translation by Frank Cole Babbitt*, London, 1928, 15 vols., reprinted 1956 (source of citation on p. v. is II, 135E).

PLUTARCH, *Plutarch's Lives, with an English translation by Bernadette Perrin*, London, 1920, 11 vols.

PRÉVOST, MARCEL, *L'automne d'une femme*, Vienna (n.d.).

RABELAIS, FRANÇOIS, *Works of Mr. Francis Rabelais* (reprint of Urquhart-Motteux translation), New York, 1932, 2 vols.

RATHER, L. J., *Disease, Life and Man, Selected Essays by Rudolf Virchow, translated and with an introduction by Lelland J. Rather*, Stanford, 1958.

ROBINSON, NICHOLAS, *A New System of the Spleen, Vapours and Hypochondriac Melancholy . . .*, London, 1729.

RYLE, GILBERT, *The Concept of Mind*, London, 1949.

SAMBURSKY, S., *The Physics of the Stoics*, New York, 1959.

SAVIOZ, RAYMOND, *Mémoires autobiographiques de Charles Bonnet de Genève*, (Diss.), Paris, 1948.

SCARAMUCCI, JOHANNE BAPTISTA, *De hydrophobo ex irae impetu tali, Acta eruditorum, IV*, Lipsiae, April, 1702.

SCHRÖDINGER, ERWIN, *Mind and Matter*, Cambridge, 1958.

Seneca, Ad Lucilium epistulae morales, with an English translation by Richard M. Gummere, London, 1925, 3 vols., reprinted 1953.

Seneca, Moral Essays, with an English translation by H. Rackham, London, 1928, 3 vols., reprinted 1958.

SMITH, W., M.D., *A Dissertation on the Nerves, containing an account, 1. of the nature of man, 2. of the nature of brutes, 3. of the nature and connection of the soul and body, 4. of the threefold life of man, 5. of the symptoms, causes and cure of all nervous diseases*, London, 1768.

STAHL, GEORG ERNST, *Negotium otiosum seu skiamachia*, Halle, 1720.

STAHL, GEORG ERNST, *Ueber den mannigfaltigen Einfluss von Gemüthsbewegungen auf den menschlichen Körper, translated by Bernward J. Gottlieb*, Sudhoff's Klassiker der Medizin, Leipzig, 1961.

STRUTH, JOSEPH, *Ars sphygmica seu pulsuum doctrina . . . a Josepho Struthio*, Basel, 1602.

SWAMMERDAM, JAN, *Biblia naturae sive historia insectorum . . .* Leydae, 1737.

SWIETEN, GERARD VAN, *Commentaria in Hermanni Boerhaavii Aphorismos*, Hildburghausen, 1754, 4 vols.

SYDENHAM, THOMAS, *The Works of Thomas Sydenham, M.D.,* *translated from the Latin edition of Dr. Greenhill by R. C.* *Latham, M.D.,* London, 1852, 2 vols.

TAYLOR, A. E., *A Commentary on Plato's Timaeus,* Oxford, 1928.

Thomae Bartholini acta medica et philosophica Hafniensia, ann. 1677, 1678, 1679, *Hafniae,* 1680, 5 vols.

TISSOT, M. (SIMON-ANDRÉ), *Essai sur les maladies des gens du monde,* 2nd ed., Lausanne, 1770.

UEBERWEG, FRIEDRICH, *Die Philosophie des Altertums, herausgegeben von Karl Praechter,* 12te Auflage, Basel/Stuttgart, 1960.

VARTANIAN, ARAM, *La Mettrie's L'Homme Machine, A Study in the Origins of an Idea,* Princeton, 1960.

WEIKARD, M., *Der philosophische Arzt, neue Auflage,* Frankfurt/M., 1798, 3 vols.

WINSLOW, JAQUES-BENIGNE, *Exposition anatomique de la structure du corps humain,* Amsterdam, 1743, 4 vols.

WRIGHT, THOMAS, *The Passions of the Minde in Generall,* London, 1621.

ZÜCKERT, J. F., *Von den Leidenschaften,* 2te Aufl., Berlin, 1768.

B. PAPERS

BIER, AUGUST, "Die Entzündung", *Arch. f. klin. Chir.,* 176: 407, 1933.

EDELSTEIN, LUDWIG, "The Relation of Ancient Philosophy to Medicine", *Bull. Hist. Med.,* 27: 299, 1952.

GERARD, R. W., "Biological Roots of Behavior", *Science,* 122: 225, 1955.

MEYER-STEINEG, THEODOR, "Hieronymus Dav. Gaub über die natürlichen Heilkräfte", *Arch. f. Gesch. d. Med.,* 15: 114, 1923.

RATHER, L. J., "G. E. Stahl's Psychological Physiology", *Bull. Hist. Med.,* Baltimore, 35: 37–49, 1961.

RUSSELL, BERTRAND, "What is Mind?" *Journal of Philosophy,* 55: 1, 1958.

SURINGAR, G. C. B. "Verval van het klinisch onderwijs na den dood van Boerhaave", etc., *Nederlandsch Tijdschrift voor Geneeskunde,* 2e Rks, 2e Jrg, 2e Afd., pp. 256–77, 1866.

WOLF, STEWART, "Disease as a Way of Life: Neural Integration in Systemic Pathology", *Perspectives in Biology and Medicine,* IV: 288, 1961.

WOLFSON, HARRY AUSTRYN, "The Internal Senses in Latin, Arabic and Hebrew Philosophic Texts", *Harvard Theological Review,* 28: 2, April, 1935.

Index

Abricossoff, Glafira, 241.

Acta medica (Hafniensis) et philosophica (Th. Bartholinus), 216, 217.

ad Lucilium epistulae morales (Seneca), 222.

Adversariorum varii argumenti (J. D. Gaub), 22.

Aeneid (Virgil), 205.

Agrippa von Nettesheim, Henry Cornelius, 225, 241.

Alcmeon, 215.

Alexander the Great, 183, 185, 241.

Alpini, Prospero, 21, 29.

Amaltheum Lexicon, 226, 231, 232, 233, 241, 242.

American Illustrated Medical Dictionary (Dorland), 226.

amor insanus (*see* love).

amulets: 174; how effective, 178, 179.

analogies: use of in teaching, 48–9.

Anatomy of Melancholy (Robert Burton), 207, 211, 219, 226, 231, 235, 236.

Ancilla to the Pre-Socratic Philosophers (Kathleen Freeman), 215.

Anfangsgründe der medizinischen Krankheitslehre (C. G. Gruner), 26.

anger, acute; harmful effects on body of —, 133–9, 183; cause of jaundice, 133, 137, 138; not always a brief madness, 134, 136; cause of dilatation of heart, 133; may damage brain, 133, 135; baneful effects on weak and ailing, 134; mechanism of harmful effects, 134, 135, 137; cause of hydrophobia, 135, 138; cause of fever, inflammation and digestive disturbances, 135; cause of urination, 136; readies body for revenge, 136; cause of hemorrhages, 137; cause of paralysis, apoplexy and sudden death, 137; cause of evacuation of bile, 137; convulsions in nursing infant due to anger of nurse, 139; cause of miscarriage, 139; most destructive and most beneficial of emotions, 181; therapeutic effects of, 183–6; cure of aphonia, 183, 184; quartan fever cured by —, 184; arthritis cured by —, 184; recalls to life temporarily those who are nearly dead, 184; effects resemble those of excessive joy, 185; doubtful value as therapy, 185, 186; in smallpox, measles and eruptive diseases, 186; Seneca on —, 221.

anger, suppressed: harmful effects of —, 139, 140; cause of death, 140; cause of fatal fever, 140.

Anticyra, 127, 129.

anxiety: bodily sources of, 55, 58, 59; treatment of madness by induced anxiety, 109, 110; in young girls, 180.

apathy (*apatheia*), Stoic: 149; not the physician's goal for his patient, 201, 202.

aphonia (*see also* loss of voice): cured by anger, 183, 184; related to retention of afterbirth, 183, 185; cured by terror, 186.

appetites (*see also* pica): healthy, conceived by the mind, 164; unusual and spontaneous —, 165.

Aquinas, x.

Archeus, 169.

Arnold, Magda, 206, 210.

Ars sphygmica seu pulsuum doctrina ... (J. Struth), 227, 230.

Attic Nights of Aulus Gellius, The (A. Gellius), 220, 225, 230, 241, 242.

Augustine, 125, 236, 240.

automata (*see also* machine, human; mechanism, mechanistic reasoning, etc.), 121.

Avicenna, 4, 213, 226, 235.

awareness: bodily activities occurring without, 50, 119; Descartes and the primacy of, 5; crucial character of, 6.

Bacon, Roger, 235.

Bartholinus, Thomas, 216, 217.

Berkeley, George, 7.

Bible, The: Galatians, 220; Job, 224.

Biblia naturae sive historica insectorum ... (Jan Swammerdam), 21, 29.

Bier, August, 23, 30.

"Biological Roots of Psychiatry" (R. W. Gerard), 25.

Black, Joseph, 22.

Bleuland, Jan B., 26.

blood: excess of — stirs up anger, ferocity and lust, 112; treatment of nymphomania by withdrawal of —, 112, 114; accumulation of — in heart and lungs due to sorrow, 142; effect of anger on circulation of —, 185.

Boas, George, v.

body: power over the mind in normal state, 51; unlimited power in disturbed states, 53; body an abstraction from whole man, 70; remedies acting on the mind may heal the — though the mind is not the cause of the bodily disease, 71; the primary object of the physician's concern, 70, 72; phantom limb phenomenon, 77; why scrutiny of — after death usually fails to explain grossly abnormal behaviour, 103, 105; danger of delay in treating bodily cause of a mental ailment, 105–7; how mismanaged by mind, 126–9; perpetual flux of —, 169; interior as well as exterior affected by emotions, 183; *domicilium mentis, domicilium animae,* 207; a prison of the mind, 42, 207.

Body and Mind (W. McDougall), 209.

Boerhaave, Hermann, 13, 19, 20, 21, 23, 28, 29, 82, 90, 117, 119, 136, 139, 154, 178, 182, 183, 191, 193, 194, 200, 213, 214, 218, 221, 222, 223, 230, 235, 236, 241, 242; medical art of reasoning *more geometrico,* 118, 119; definition of disease, 119; on diuresis in hysteria and hypochondria, 191; how emotions in general disturb secretion, 191; cure of mental disturbances by induced terror, 193; on submersion therapy, 193.

Boerhaave, Abraham Kaau-, 18, 26.

Boethius, Hector, 216.

bond: between mind and body, 34, 204.

Bonnet, Charles, 13, 218.

Borelli, 121.

Borrichius, Olaus (Ole Borch), 100, 103, 184, 187, 217, 241.

Boyle, Robert, 3, 120, 188, 192, 209, 219, 233, 242.

Bremond, Henri, 231.

Bright, Timothy, 236.

Buchanan, Scott, 231.

Bugati, 104.

Burton, Robert, 207, 211, 226, 231, 235, 236, 242.

Cabanis, Pierre Jean George, 10, 26.

Caligula, 55, 58.

cancer: influenced by emotions, 17; onset and recurrence influenced by fear and sorrow, 147.

cannibalism: in pregnant women, 101; in Scottish girl, 102, 118.

Cannon, Walter, 208.

Cantica . . . (Avicenna), 213.

Canus Julius, 54, 57, 118, 209.

Carrère, Joseph, 121, 219.

Catherine the Great, 18, 242.

cause: equivocal character of psychic factors as initiators of somatic disease, 2, 3; emotional excess as — of bodily disease, 8; remote — of hysteria a mental disturbance (Sydenham), 189; ultimate —s not the physician's concern, 73, 104, 119; predisposing and occasional —s, 105.

Cavendish, Henry, 22.

Celsus, 36, 133, 207.

Charmides (Plato), 190, 214, 231.

charms: 174; how effective, 178, 179, 184; Burton on, 235; Bacon on, 235.

Chauvet, Emmanuel, 206.

chlorosis, 150.

Cicero, Marcus Tullius, 14, 34, 39, 45, 56, 60, 62; inversion of his views by Gaub, 90, 95, 123; on parts of the mind, 124; *Tusculan Disputations* quoted by Gaub, 124, 131, 133, 139, 157–9, 200, 205, 207, 208–9, 214, 216, 220, 221, 229, 230, 236.

Cimetière marin, Le (Valéry), 25.

Circulation of the Blood and Other Writings, The (William Harvey), 224.

clockwork: men and animals seen as, 121.

coction, 170.

Collected Dialogues, The (Plato), 231.

Collections des thèses soutenues a l'école de Montpellier . . ., 222.

Collingwood, R. G., 211.

Commentaria in Hermanni Boerhaavii aphorismos (Gerard van Swieten), 221.

Commentary on Plato's Timaeus, A (A. E. Taylor), 210, 215.

complexio (*see also* temperament, mixture, krasis), 213.

259

computer, humanoid, 5.
Concept of Mind, The (Gilbert Ryle), 25.
consensus (see also sympathy), 35, 205.
Considérations politiques sur les coups d'état (Gabriel Naudé), 217.
Cornaro, Luigi, 158, 160, 231.
Corp, Dr. — of Bath, 137, 139, 143, 145, 146, 147, 153, 175, 176, 177, 178, 182, 185, 186, 193, 194, 222, 224, 225, 226, 229, 234, 235, 241, 242.
Cratylus (Plato), 207.
Croesus, 185, 186.
Coup d'œil sur les révolutions et sur la réforme de la médecine (P. J. G. Cabanis), 26.
courage: physiological determinants of —, 54, 55, 57, 58.
custom: tyranny of —, 197.
Damenkrankheit, 200.
Danto, Arthur, 25.
Daremberg, Charles H., 114; on Galen's misunderstanding of Aristotle, 206, 217.
"Dass die Vermögen der Seele eine Folge der Mischungen des Körpers sind" (Erika Hauke), 206.
De anima (Avicenna), 235.
De Brunn, 29.
De Moor, Bartholomew, 19.
De humoribus (pseudo-Galenical), 233.
De hydrophobo ex irae impetu tali (J. B. Scaramucci), 223.
"De l'influence des passions sur l'économie animale, considérée dans les quatre âges de la vie" (Raimund Laroque), 222.
De medica historia mirabili (Marcellus Donatus), 216.
De medicina (Celsus), 207, 222.
De morbis animi (B. Perdulcis or Pardoux), 216, 217, 228.
De occulta philosophia . . . (H. C. Agrippa von Nettesheim), 225.
De oratore (Cicero), 221.
De Peiresc, N. F., 179, 180.
De placitis Hippocratis et Platonis . . . (C. Galen), 220.
De praesagienda vita et morti aegrotatium libri septem . . . (P. Alpini), 29.
death: apparently due to injury but in reality due to emotional disturbance, 134.
Democritus (pseudo) cited: v., 20, 36, 37, 78, 84, 174, 178, 214.
Der Wahnsinn: Geschichte der abendländischen Psychopathologie (W. Leibbrand and A. Wettley), 231.
Descartes, René: 1, 3, 4; on primacy of awareness, 5; on separation of mind and body, 7, 8, 25, 40, 47; definition of thought, 52; how bodily changes cause emotions and not vice versa, 57; role of pineal gland, 57; conflict between higher and lower parts of mind actually a conflict between mind and body via the pineal gland, 57, 124; emotions prepare body for fight or flight, 57, 208, 59; ambiguities in his theory of the

emotions, 63, 64; dependence of mind on temperament and state of
bodily organs, 74, 81, 96; —, Galen and Gaub on the medical management of the mind, 113, 117, 118, 119; human body compared to
piece of clockwork, 121, 125, 132, 133; on location of mind, 206, 210,
211, 212, 214, 219–22, 224, 225, 236, 239; his view of the emotions,
14, 15.

erotomania (*see* love).

Essai sur les maladies des gens du monde (M. Tissot), 221.

Essais, texte établi et annoté par Albert Thibaudet (Montaigne), 209.

Essay on the Changes Produced in the Body by the Operations of the Mind, An (Corp), 222.

euthanasia: 158; definition of, 160.

experiment: use of, 111.

Exposition anatomique de la structure du corps humain (J.-B. Winslow), 210.

faith: effects of patient's — in physician, 174, 178.

Fasch, Augustin, 120, 219.

fashions: harmful effects of, 128, 129, 130.

Faust (J. W. von Goethe), 25.

feelings, 7.

Feigl, Herbert, 210.

Feuchtersleben, Ernst von, 24, 30.

fever: effects of, 55, 59, 112; usually beneficial, 170, 171.

fibers: elementary, how generated (Gaub), 20.

force of habit: determining recurrence of nervous diseases, 194.

Forcellini, 218.

Fragmente der Vorsokratiker, Griechisch und Deutsch, Die (Hermann Diels), 205.

Francke, August Hermann, 19, 27.

"Free Inquiry into the Vulgarly Received Notion of Nature, A" (Robert Boyle), 219.

free will, 13, 39.

Freeman, Kathleen, 215.

Frerichs, Friedrich Theodor, 223.

Friedreich, J. B., 233.

Fuchs, Robert, 214, 215, 226.

function: two orders of, 49, 52.

"G. E. Stahl's Psychological Physiology" (L. J. Rather), 25, 207.

Gaius Caesar, 54.

Galen: 10, 14, 16; Gaub's use of — as a source, 14; on the emotions as causes of bodily disease, 16; persistence of Galenical tradition, 17; indirectly cited by Gaub, 79; effects of body on mind, 36, 84, 85; title of Galenical essay on temperaments indirectly cited by Gaub, 85, 87; cited by Gaub, 92; on the temperaments as states of imbalance, 94, 95; on *sophrosynê*, 62, 63, 82, 96, 97, 108, 113, 114, 117, 150, 151, 159, 181; Daremberg and Chauvet on —, 206; 208, 209, 212, 213, 215, 217, 220, 226, 227, 229, 230, 231, 233, 241.

ganscho (ganja, cannabis activa): effects of, 112, 114.

Gassendi, Pierre, 179, 180, 235.

Gaub, Christoph, 18.

Gaub, Constantia, 20.

hemorrhage: in emotional disturbances (*see* anger, terror), mechanism of, 185.

hexis, Stoic philosophers on, 205.

"Hieronymus Dav. Gaub über die natürlichen Heilkräfte" (T. Meyer-Steineg), 30.

Hippocrates, 10, 36, 60, 62; cited by Gaub, 111, 113, 118, 139, 150, 151, 169, 180, 185, 186, 196, 209, 214, 215, 232, 235, 239.

Hippocrates, with an English translation by W. H. S. Jones, 217.

Hippocratic Oath, The (Ludwig Edelstein), 215.

Histoire de la psychologie de l'antiquité à nos jours (F. Louis-Mueller), 220.

Histore littéraire du sentiment religieux en France (H. Bremond), 231.

History of Biology . . ., The (Eric Nordenskiöld), 29.

history of medicine, aim of, x, xi.

History of the Scots (H. Boethius), 216.

Hoffmann, Friedrich H., 222.

Hofkrankheit, 200.

Holland, Philip, 145, 147, 152, 193, 225, 226, 227.

homesickness: 143, 149, 150; sufferers from — revived by hope, 174, 175; frequent in Switzerland, 175; may lead to death, 175; case history of, 175–6; causes and mechanism of, 176, 177; bodily symptoms of, 177; Verhovitz on, 233; Larrey on, 234.

hope: beneficial effects of, 173, 177, 178; explains cures of quacks, 174; delays death, 174; mechanism of action, 175; cure of homesickness, 175; should be maintained to the last, 178; aids cure of certain fevers, 178; remains delusively high in consumption, 178.

Horace, 136, 222.

hormen (*see* enormôn).

Hume, David, 8, 26, 47, 48, 207.

humors: effect of fever in hastening circulation of, 112; corruption of — by anger, 134, 135, 138, 139; emotional changes of — due to power of common sensorium, 139; changes induced by grief, 141; disturbed by sorrow, 142; movement of — accelerated by hope, 174, 178; altered by homesickness, 177; altered by emotions, 8, 239; circuit of — weakened by emotional apathy, 201.

Hunter, Richard, 219, 241, 242.

hydrophobia: caused by acute anger, 135, 138.

hypochondria: cured by terror, 187; Sydenham on —, 189–90 (*see also* hysteria).

hysteria: associated with corruption of humors, 134; hysterical convulsions caused by grief, terror or anger, 143, 182; in love-sickness, 152; Galenical explanation of, 185; hysterical aphonia cured by terror, 186; Sydenham on, 189–90; diuresis in —, 190, 191; *globus hystericus* in, 191; (*see also* hypochondria); "chameleon of diseases ', 190.

ibn Ishāq (Joannitius), 16, 213.

idea: definition of (Boas), v.; transformation of — into corporeal exemplar, 178, 179.

illness: of mind often caused by body, 71; of body often caused by mind, 71.
imagination: corporeal aspect of, 77; power to produce disease, 17, 178, 179.
impetum faciens, 139.
incantations, how effective, 178.
inheritance, transmission of behavioral traits via, 101.
instinct: of beasts sometimes more reliable than human reason, 126, 129; defined as quasi-rational, 161; blind, 167.
Institutiones medicae, . . . (H. Boerhaave), 213, 218, 236.
Institutiones pathologiae medicinalis (J. D. Gaub), 23, 167, 205, 209, 210, 211, 212, 213, 215, 217, 221, 222, 223, 224, 225, 232.
intemperance (*see* temperance).
"Internal Senses in Latin, Arabic and Hebrew Philosophic Texts" (H. A. Wolfson), 213.
Introducción Histórica al Estudio de la Patología Psicosomática (P. Lain-Entralgo), 26.
irritability, and the *enormôn*, 66.
Isagoge ad tegni Galeni (Joannitius, ibn Ishāq), 16, 213.
isotheos, 111, 113.
Jaeger, Werner, 214.
James, William, 6, 25.
jaundice: caused by acute anger, 133, 136, 138; caused by terror, 145.
Jauregg, Julius Wagner von, 230.
Joannitius (ibn Ishāq), 16, 212, 213.
Johannis Gaubii epistola problematica . . . ad virum clarissimum Fredericum Ruyschium (Joan Gaub), 27.
joy: unrestrained, effects of, 148, 152–4; cause of fever, 153; cause of temporary insanity, 153; sudden death in, 154; beneficial effect of joy, 180.
Juncker, Johann, 146, 152, 154, 193, 225, 227, 230, 242.
Juvenal, 212.
King Ferdinand, 141.
King John of Hungary, 141.
kleptomania, 104, 118 (*see also* pregnancy).
Klinik der Leberkrankheiten (T. Frerichs), 223.
Körperbau und Charakter (E. Kretschmer), 215.
Koestler, Arthur, 206.
krasis: 205, 206; analogy with *sôphrosynê*, 215 (*see also* temperament).
Kretschmer, Ernst, 215.
Krumbhaar, E. B., 30.
Kühn, C. G., 108, 209, 215, 217, 241.
L'automne d'une femme (Marcel Prévost), 227.
L'Hystérie aux XVIIe et XVIIIe siècles (G. Abricossoff), 241.
La Curación por la Palabra en la Antigüedad Clásica (P. Lain-Entralgo), 231.
La Mettrie, Julien, 13, 66; Gaub on —, 115, 116; use of Gaub's lecture in *Man a Machine*, 117, 118, 121.

La Mettrie's L'Homme Machine, *A Study in the Origins of an Idea* (A. Vartanian), 218.

Laehr, Heinrich, 26, 220.

Lain-Entralgo, Pedro, 15, 16, 26, 231.

Laroque, Raimund, 137, 147, 152, 191, 222, 226, 227.

Larrey, Baron Dominique Jean, 234.

laughter (see also joy): effects of extravagant, 148.

Lavoisier, Antoine, 22.

Lebenswelt, 9.

Leibbrand, Werner, 231, 252.

Leibniz, Gottfried Wilhelm, 11, 42, 46, 47, 121, 154, 207, 212, 219.

Lemnius, Levine, 213, 232.

Libellus de methodo concinnandi formulas medicamentorum . . . (J. D. Gaub), 29.

Liber canonis . . . (Avicenna), 213.

life: social contract of, 38; disease as life under abnormal conditions, 23.

Literatur der Psychiatrie, Neurologie und Psychologie im 18 ten Jahrhundert, Die (H. Laehr), 26, 220.

Littré, Émile, 209, 212, 214, 217, 235.

Lives of Eminent Philosophers (Diogenes Laertius), 234.

loss of voice, due to fear or terror, 144, 146.

Louis-Mueller, Fernand, 220.

love: as a cause of mental derangement, 109; harmful effects of unrequited —, 149–52; difficulty of detecting love-sickness, 150; diagnosed by Hippocrates, Erasistratus, Galen, 150; green-sickness in , 150, 152; changes induced in pulse, 151; a plague to body and mind, 152; heartbreak in, 152; a cause of insanity, 152; nymphomania in, 152; in restoring body heat, 179, 180; pathology and therapy of (Perdulcis), 227–9.

Lovejoy, Arthur O., 25.

machine: human and animal (*see also* La Mettrie, mechanism, mechanistic reasoning): criteria for distinguishing men from machines, 5; ghost in the machine, 6; Boerhaave on, 120; Boyle on, 3, 120; Fasch on, 120; Smith on, 121; consequences of belief that animals are machines, 122.

machine: needed to inspire terror in the insane, 187.

Maine de Biran, Reformer of Empiricism (P. P. Hallie), 207.

mal de cour (*see Hofkrankheit*).

maladie des dames à quarante ans (*see Damenkrankheit*).

maladie du pays (*see also* homesickness), 176.

Man a Machine (*see* La Mettrie, Julien).

materia peccans, 170.

Macalpine, Ida, 219, 241, 242.

McDougall, William, 63, 209.

mechanism (*see also* La Mettrie): crises of disease and the human mechanism, 120; when acceptable, 120, 121; Leibniz on, 121, 219; Carrère on, 121; Borelli on, 121.

mechanistic reasoning: Boerhaave on its applicability to medicine, 119.

Meckel, J. F., 29.

medicaments: abuse of, 128, 129; different effects of, 156.

medicine: perennial concern of Western medicine with mind-body relationships, x, 1, 9; psychosomatic medicine no novelty, x; double aspect of
   psychosomatic medicine (Lain-Entralgo), 16.

Medicina rationalis systematica (Friedrich H. Hoffmann), 222.

melancholy, 151.

Mémoires autobiographiques de Charles Bonnet de Genève (R. Savioz), 218.

memory: corporeal aspect of, 77; weakening of — by blood loss, 112, 113.

*"Mental " and the "Physical " in Concepts, Theories, and the Mind–Body
   Problem, The* (Herbert Feigl), 210.

Mercer, Graemius, 147, 226.

Merleau-Ponty, Maurice, 5, 25, 84, 214.

Metaphysics (R. G. Collingwood), 211.

metus (see terror).

Meyer-Steineg, Theodor, 23, 30.

Milton, John, 233.

mind: meaning of, since Descartes, 6, 7; cannot be an efficient cause in a
   physical system, 6; as a quasi-material substance, 35; cannot be managed
   without attending to body, 35, 203; limits of power over body in normal
   state, 50, 54; unlimited power over body in disturbed states, 53;
   effects of gout and colic on —, 54; relation to part of nervous system
   superintending senses and voluntary movement, 65; — an abstraction
   from whole man, 70; remedies acting on the body may heal a —
   either ailing on its own account or due to bodily derangement, 71;
   legitimacy of physician's concern with the —, 71–3, 80; physicians
   vs. philosophers in the care of the —, 73, 74, 202, 203; power of
   bodily organs to deceive —, 77; effects of overstraining the —,
   75, 82, 83; only the physician can cure diseases of the — originating in
   the body, 90; differences in men's —s due to differences in their
   temperaments, 94; corruption of — of infant by milk of wet-nurse, 102,
   104; difficulty of determining whether — is suffering on its own
   account or on that of the body, 105, 106; physician can restore — by
   treating body, 119; rational and irrational parts of, 122–5; *psychê, thymos*
   and *epithymia*, 124; should check her own *enormôn*, 130; power to
   control body, according to Descartes, 132; power of — over body
   equally capable of good or ill effects, 155, 156; part of divine —, 154,
   158; concern for afflicted body, 163, 169; as sole cause of bodily complaints, 182.

Mind and Body (P. Lain-Entralgo), 26.

Mind and Matter (E. Schrödinger), 25.

mind–body problem: a dilemma, 4, 5; antedates Cartesianism, 7, 8; insoluble
   character of, 48, 51; philosophical distinguished from physiological, 2,
   51, 69, 123.

mind–body interaction: in the normal state, 48–52; Gaub's inability to explain its basis, 48; constraining laws of, 49; power of body over mind greater than that of mind over body, 51; in states of disturbance, 53; reverberative character of disturbances of, 55, 56; speed of, 61; mechanism of interaction in emotional disturbances, 68–70; in overstrain of the mind, 83; according to Stahl, 181, 182; according to Valangin, 182; according to Boerhaave, 183; according to Zückert, 182; according to Smith, 182; pineal gland or body as site of, 8.

mixture, 34, 35, 205, 206 (*see also* krasis).

molimina: 168; described, 169.

Montaigne, Michael de, 141, 142, 153, 209, 224, 229, 230.

Moral Essays (Seneca), 221.

more geometrico (*see* mechanistic reasoning).

Morgagni, Giovanni Battista, 23, 29, 137, 138, 222, 223.

Movement of the Heart and Blood (Harvey/Franklin), 240.

Murray, Margaret H., 217.

Natural History of the Soul (Julien La Mettrie), 118.

nature: limits of human understanding of, 116; the true physician of disease, 130; healing powers of, 13, 161–72; Gaub's idea of nature, 167, 168; disease as a "contest of nature", 168; the physician of diseases, 168; not infallible, 168; defensive efforts may be worse than the disease, 169.

Naudé, Gabriel, 112, 114, 217.

Negotium otiosum seu skiamachia (G. W. Leibniz), 219.

nêpenthe: 112; Daremberg on, 114.

nervous system (see also mind): 65, 124; tone restored by hope, 174; energized by hope, 177; and mental diseases, 182; involved in all diseases, 182; and chronic disease, 183; hysteria and hypochondria as diseases of the — (Sydenham), 189.

Neurophysiological Basis of Mind, The (John Eccles), 25, 208.

New System of the Spleen, Vapours and Hypochondriac Melancholy . . ., A (N. Robinson), 241.

Niobe, transformation by grief, 141, 142.

non-naturals: in relation to the *enormôn* of the body, 78, 79, 81, 82, 84; Galen and the non-naturals, 82; Boerhaave and the —, 82, 113; abuse of, 127, 129, 149; Boyle on the —, 192, 199; origin of doctrine of, 212, 213; doctrine of, 16, 17; importance in prolonging life, 21, 38.

Nordenskiöld, Eric, 29.

nosimanias, 176 (*see also* homesickness).

nostalgia (*see also* homesickness): 175; origin of term, 176.

nymphomania (*see also* love, disease of virgins): 152; Hippocratic cure of, 180.

Observationes circa hominem et ejusque morbos (F. M. van Helmont), 217.

Observationum medicarum . . . (P. Salmuth), 242.

Observationum medicarum rararum, . . . (Schenck von Grafenberg), 216.

Observationum physico-medicarum libri tres (J. N. Pechlin), 222.

observer (Einsteinian), 6.

psychosomatic medicine: permissibility of applying this term to Gaub's work, 10 (*see also* medicine, mind–body interaction, etc.).

pulse: in love-sickness, 151; of a person, 10; effects of various emotions on (Struth), 226–7.

Puschmann's Handbuch der Geschichte der Medizin (art. Robert Fuchs), 214, 215.

Pythagoras, 35, 37, 79, 85, 96, 97, 123.

Quod animalia bruta saepe ratione utantur melius homine (Rorarius), 220.

Quod animi mores corporis temperamenta sequantur (Galen), 97.

Rabelais, Francis, 230.

Ramspeck, J. C., 29.

Rather, Lelland Joseph, 25, 29, 207, 210.

Recueil de mémoires de chirurgie (D. J. Larrey), 234.

"Relations of Ancient Philosophy to Medicine, The" (Ludwig Edelstein), 212.

remedies (see also medicaments): appetites in illness may point to remedies needed, 164, 165; faith in physician increases power of, 174; insufficiency of — with respect to diseases of mind, 198.

res cogitans and *res extensa*, 8, 11.

Revolt against Dualism, The (A. O. Lovejoy), 25.

Rhine, J. B., 4.

Richardson, Dr., 187, 192, 227.

right reason: 116, 131; corporeal benefits of, 154, 156.

Robinson, Nicholas, 184, 241.

Rorarius, 220.

Russell, Bertrand, 219.

Ruysch, Frederick, 27.

Ryle, Gilbert, 6, 25, 219.

Salmuth, Philipp, 192, 242.

Sambursky, S., 205.

Savioz, Raymond, 218.

Scaramucci, Johanne Baptista, 138, 223.

Sceptical Chymist, The (Robert Boyle), 209.

Schenck von Grafenberg, 104, 216.

Schrödinger, Erwin, 25.

Schwarz, Oswald, 231.

Seats and Causes of Diseases Investigated by Anatomy, The (J. B. Morgagni), 222.

Seneca, 57, 133, 138, 200, 221, 222.

senses, internal or interior, 77, 83.

sleep, prolonged (*see* Endymion's sleep).

Sleepwalkers, The (A. Koestler), 206.

Smith, W., M.D., 143, 147, 182, 191, 219, 224, 226, 235, 242.

Socrates, 90, 160, 207.

sôphrosynê (*see also* temperance and temperaments): as temperance of mind according to Cicero, 95; rooted in bodily *krasis*, 97, 113; Galen on, 159; analogy with *krasis*, 215.

sorrow (*see* grief).

soul: 101; unity of — according to Augustine, 125 (*see also psychê*).

Specimen inaugurale medicum exhibens ideam generalem solidarum corporis humani partium . . . (J. D. Gaub), 27.

Speeches, The (Cicero), 205.

spirit, human: fallibility of, 126, 129.

Spirit of disease . . ., *The* (F. M. van Helmont), 242.

Stahl, Georg Ernst, 22, 25, 46, 57, 121, 140, 181, 193, 207, 219, 224, 225, 235, 242.

Struth, Joseph, 226, 227, 230.

submersion therapy: in the treatment of mental derangement, 109, 110, 187, 191, 192.

suppuration: beneficial character of, 170.

Suringar, G. C. B., 26, 28, 29.

Swammerdam, Jan, 21, 29.

Swieten, Gerard van, 129, 178, 221.

Sydenham, Thomas, 189, 190, 191, 241.

sympathy (*see also* harmony) of body and mind, 182, 191, 205.

sympathetic cures, physiological explanation of, 192.

Taprell, J., ix.

Taylor, A. E., 63, 97, 210, 215.

tears: beneficial effect of — in sorrow, 142, 143; no disgrace in, 142.

temperament: 85–97; variability of, 85, 87; and character, 85; seat of diversity of —s in body, 86; correlation with character by Galen, 87; classification and description of, 88–90; imbalance of —s according to Gaub, 90; according to Galen, 94, 95; may be modified by physician, 91, 92; variety of temperaments neglected by the physician, 92, 93; and the four elements, 97; and the four seasons, 97; frequently altered by mind, 181, 182; a modern view of, 215; influence on mind exerted by, 14.

temperance (*see also* temperament): Cicero on, 95; intemperance of mind, 148; bodily factors favor intemperance, 148, 149; Cicero and Galen on, 159, 160; two meanings of intemperance, 159.

terror (and fear): 143–7; the most violent of the emotions, 143; list of effects attributed to —, 144; effect on the imagination in pregnancy, 144; loss of sphincter control in —, 144, 145, 147; abortion induced by—, 145; fear and terror differentiated, 145; effect on nervous system, 145; a case of death due to chronic fear, 145; physiological effects of —, 146; sudden death due to —, 146; discharge of semen in —, 147; suppression of lactation and menstruation in—, 147; most destructive and most beneficial of the emotions, 181; effects resemble those of anger, 185; as therapy, 186–94; cure of aphonia, 186; cure of fever by —, 187, 192, 194; hypochondria cured by —, 187; employed against rabies, 187, 192;

MADE AND PRINTED IN GREAT BRITAIN BY WILLIAM CLOWES AND SONS LIMITED, LONDON AND BECCLES